Self-assessment picture tests

Avian
Medicin

Related titles published in Mosby's Testing series include:

Cardiology
Clinical Dermatology
Clinical Infectious Disease
Clinical Medicine
Clinical Neurology
Clinical Surgery
Dermatology
Ear, Nose and Throat
Embryology, 2nd Edition
Endocrinology, 2nd Edition
Gastroenterology, 2nd Edition
Hematology
Human Histology
Human Anatomy

Hypertension
Infectious Diseases
Injury in Sport
Medicine:
  Vols 1–4
Oral Medicine
Orthopaedics
Otolaryngology
Paediatrics
Pathology
Renal Disease
Rheumatology
Sexually Transmitted Diseases
Urology

Self-assessment picture tests
Avian
Medicine

Brian H. Coles
BVSc, MRCVS, Dip ECAMS
RCVS Specialist in Zoo and Wildlife Medicine (Avian)
Chester, United Kingdom

Maria E. Krautwald-Junghanns
Dr Med Vet, Dr Med Vet habil, Dip ECAMS
Institute for Avian and Reptile Diseases
University of Giessen, Germany

Contributor
Thomas J. Herrman
Dr Med Vet
Institute for Avian and Reptile Diseases
University of Giessen, Germany

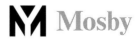
Mosby

St. Louis Baltimore Boston Carlsbad Chicago Minneapolis New York Philadelphia Portland
London Milan Sydney Tokyo Toronto

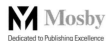
Mosby
Dedicated to Publishing Excellence

Publisher: John A. Schrefer
Executive Editor: Linda L. Duncan
Senior Developmental Editor: Teri Merchant
Project Manager: Mark Spann
Senior Production Editor: Beth Hayes
Book Design Manager: Judi Lang
Manufacturing Manager: Debbie LaRocca
Senior Composition Specialist: Peggy Hill

Lithography/color film by Top Graphics
Printing/binding by Walsworth Press, Inc.

Mosby, Inc.
11830 Westline Industrial Drive
St. Louis, Missouri 63146

Library of Congress Cataloging-in-Publication Data
Coles, B. H. (Brian H.)
   Self-assessment picture tests : avian medicine / Brian H. Coles &
Maria E. Krautwald–Junghanns.
         p.   cm.
   Includes bibliographical references.
   ISBN 0-7234-3008-X
   1. Avian medicine--Outlines, syllabi, etc. 2. Avian medicine–
-Examinations, questions, etc.   I. Krautwald, Maria-Elisabeth.
   SF994.C65   1998   98-31100
   636.5ı08—dc21   CIP

99   00   01   02   03   /   9   8   7   6   5   4   3   2   1

Preface

The purpose of this book is to present a selection of photographs of avian medical and surgical conditions likely to be seen by colleagues in general, avian, or zoologic practice, against which veterinarians can test their knowledge. As broad a range of species and clinical cases as possible has been prepared so that the whole field of avian medicine is covered. The reader is also presented with a few selected questions on the taxonomy and natural history of a species, because sometimes a knowledge of this is necessary in making a definitive diagnosis.

No attempt has been made to arrange the cases in any sort of system of disease or species order; rather they are presented at random, in much the same way as they would be to the clinician in the field. In this way the practicing veterinarian must constantly switch his or her thinking from one disease or body system to another and then later come back to that part of clinical medicine, thereby reinforcing what has been previously learned.

Brian H. Coles
Maria E. Krautwald-Junghanns

Acknowledgments

The authors are indebted to Sara Postlethwaite, who provided a great deal of secretarial help, to Dr. Ineke Westerhof for advice on Fig. 164, and to the following colleagues for the use of their slides: Dr. Baker (Fig. 67), Dr. Balks (Figs. 108, 150, 160, 161, 167, 175, and 205), Dr. Neumann (Figs. 99, 101, 109, 110, 119, and 158), Dr. Piera de Palma (Fig. 224), and Professor Rautenfeld (Fig. 59). Finally, the authors are grateful for the considerable forbearance shown by their respective spouses during the preparation of this work.

Contents

Self-assessment picture tests

Avian
Medicine

Questions

→ **1 a & b**
(a) What is the species or the type of these two birds?
(b) What factors are responsible for the color of feathers?
(c) How can disease affect the color of plumage?

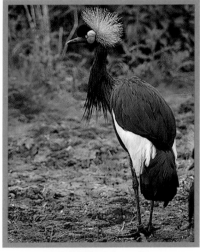

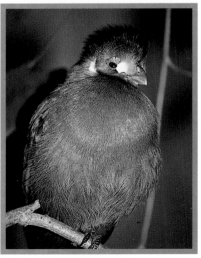

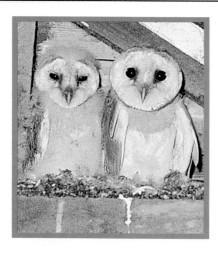

← **2**

This picture shows two young owls.
(a) To which species do they belong?
(b) These fledglings are in their first molt. Why are they at slightly different stages of molt?
(c) What do you know about normal molting in birds?
(d) When does it occur and what factors influence it?

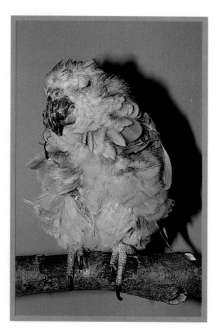

← **3**

This Amazon parrot was presented with obviously abnormal plumage and apathy.
(a) What diagnostic procedures would you suggest?
(b) How would you treat the abnormal feathering?

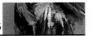

→ 4

This is the foot of a blackbird *(Turdus merula)* exhibiting hyperkeratosis.

(a) In what species of birds is this condition seen?

(b) How common is it and what is its etiology?

(c) Is it of any clinical significance?

(d) How would you treat this condition?

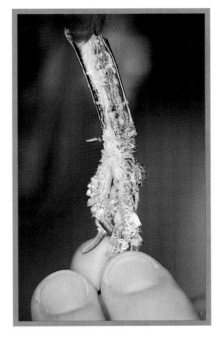

→ 5

This is the foot of a wild common buzzard *(Buteo buteo)* that presented with necrosis of the lower part of the leg.

(a) What is the likely etiology of this lesion?

(b) How may this condition affect a bird's activities?

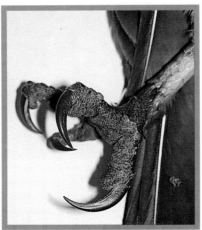

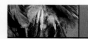

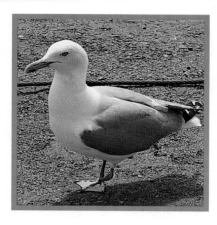

← 6

This mature herring gull *(Larus argentatus)* has lost its left foot below the tarsometatarsal joint.
(a) How do you think this has happened?
(b) What are the prospects for its survival in the wild?

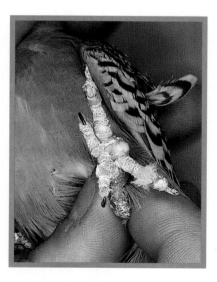

← 7

This is the foot of a budgerigar *(Melopsittacus undulatus)* that presented with a history of sitting straddle-legged on its perch and having difficulty gripping the perch.
(a) What is your diagnosis?
(b) What do you know about this condition?
(c) What line of treatment can be adopted?

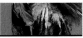

→ **8**

This fecal sample was found in an aviary containing some recently imported New World psittacine birds. Several birds had died acutely within the previous 2 days. Other clinical signs included anorexia and apathy. These birds had been housed in the same building as a group of imported conures.

(a) What disease do you suspect?
(b) How would you confirm your diagnosis?
(c) How would you treat the flock?

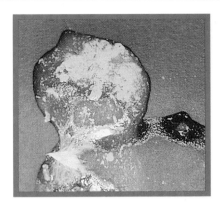

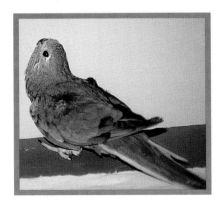

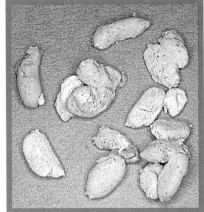

↑ **9, 10**

Several *Neophema* parrots *(Neophema pulchella)* exhibit central nervous system signs (i.e., opisthotonos and torticollis). They also have passed abnormal, light-colored, waxy stools, which with Lugol's iodine gave a strong blue positive reaction for starch.

(a) What is this disease?
(b) How should you deal with an outbreak?

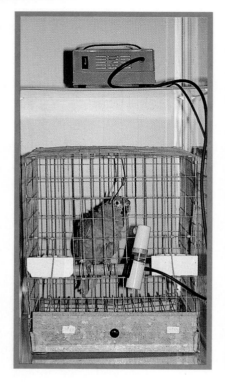

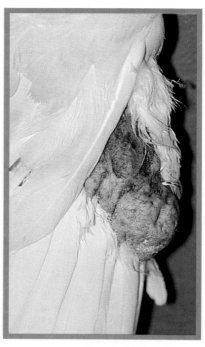

↑ **11**
This red lored Amazon parrot
(Amazona autummalis) is receiving
intensive treatment in a hospital
cage. What do you know about the
principles and application of
nebulization therapy?

↑ **12**
This is the wing of a cockatoo
with a progressively enlarging
skin lesion. How would you
arrive at a diagnosis?

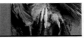

→ **13**

You are asked by the owner of this bird what is wrong with the plumage of which this feather is an example.

(a) What is the cause of this condition?

(b) How would you investigate the problem?

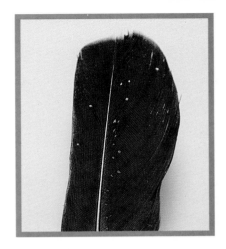

→ **14**

This magnified view of a parasite (approximately 3 mm in normal body size) was found on a wild bird.

(a) What is this parasite?

(b) On what species of wild birds are they commonly found?

(c) Are they of any clinical significance?

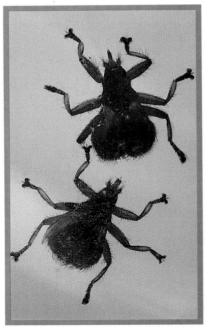

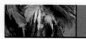

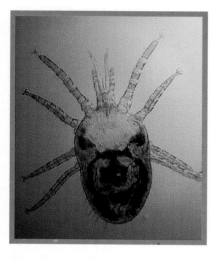

← 15
This invertebrate was recovered from the inside of a hospital cage shortly after a dying wild sparrowhawk *(Accipiter nisus)* had been placed inside for intensive therapy. As the bird died, innumerable moving black specks were found, which on microscopical examination proved to be the parasite illustrated.
(a) What is this parasite?
(b) Comment on the sudden invasion of the glass cage.
(c) What is the clinical significance of this parasite?
(d) On what species of birds does it occur?

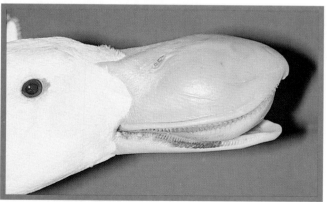

↑ 16
This goose presented with anorexia resulting from a markedly swollen upper beak and with obvious hyperthermia.
(a) What is the likely cause of these symptoms?
(b) How would you treat this bird and what is the prognosis?

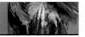

→ **17**

(a) What is this bird's species?

(b) Is its beak normal? Is it possible to say what is the sex of this bird?

(c) Can you see any lesions? What is a possible cause of these lesions?

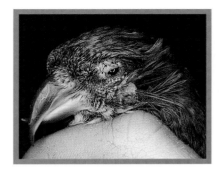

→ **18**

(a) Of what species is this bird a member?

(b) Is the feathering on its head normal? Can you see any lesions on this bird?

(c) What is the prognosis for this particular specimen?

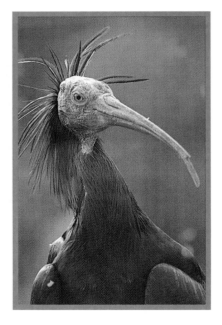

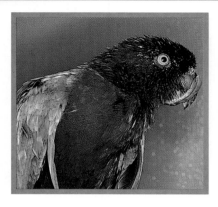

← 19

This red shining parrot *(Prosopeia tabuensis)* from Fiji has a grossly overgrown mandibular beak, which has deviated to one side of the upper, or maxillary, beak.
(a) How could this have occurred?
(b) Can anything be done to alleviate this condition?

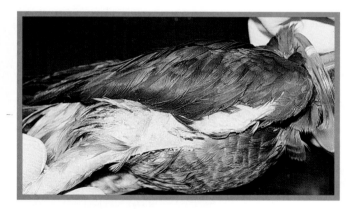

↑ 20

This illustration shows the flank of an African grey parrot *(Psittacus erithacus)* with an area of feather loss and scaly skin. A heavy infection of *Aspergillus* sp. was isolated from this case.
(a) What other clinical signs are often seen after infection with this microorganism?
(b) What do you know about other common mycotic infections of the skin of birds?
(c) How would you confirm your diagnosis?
(d) What therapy would you suggest?

→ 21

This young turquoise parrot
(Neophema pulchella) showed a
sudden symmetric loss of most of
the main wing and tail flight
feathers.
(a) What condition does this
    suggest?
(b) What do you know about its
    pathology?
(c) Is there any treatment?
(d) What routine would you
    suggest for eliminating the
    condition from an aviary?

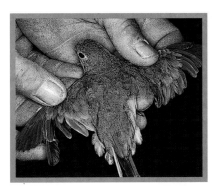

→ 22

This lesser sulphur crested cockatoo
(Cacatua sulphurea) presented with
feather loss over the whole body.
There was no sign of pruritus.
(a) What is your tentative
    diagnosis?
(b) What are the typical clinical
    signs and the course of this
    disease?

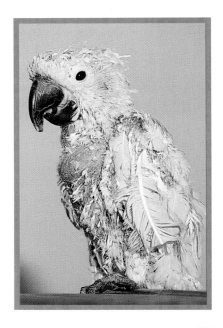

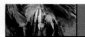

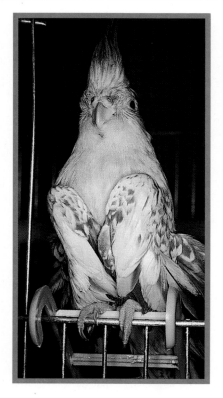

← **23**

This Lutino cockatiel *(Nymphicus hollandicus)* presented with both wings cramped in an abnormal position quite stiffly over the pectoral muscles. Physical examination showed that flexion and extension of all the joints in the wings was considerably reduced. The bird was able to perch and moved around on its legs and was feeding normally.

(a) What is your presumptive diagnosis?
(b) How would you confirm your diagnosis?
(c) What do you know about this condition?

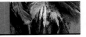
➜ **24**

This Canada goose *(Branta canadensis)* has an abnormality involving the feathers of both wings.

(a) What is the likely cause?
(b) How would you investigate the problem?
(c) Can anything be done to alleviate this condition?

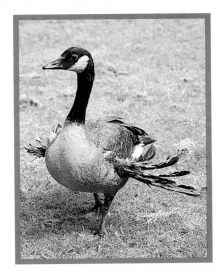

➜ **25**

(a) Is the beak of this peregrine falcon *(Falco peregrinus)* normal?
(b) If not, what is the etiology of this condition?
(c) What therapeutic measures should be carried out?

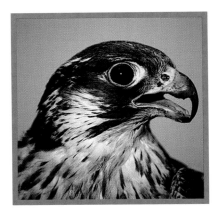

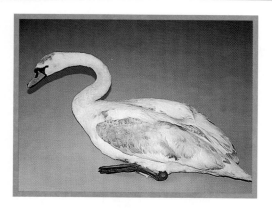

↑ 26

This subadult mute swan *(Cygnus olor)* is unable to stand and cannot raise its head. What are your differential diagnoses? What do you know of the principal conditions likely to be involved? How would you confirm your tentative diagnosis?

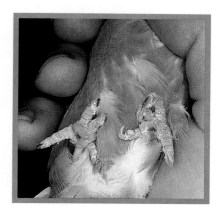

← 27

The feet of this budgerigar *(Melopsittacus undulatus)* have pododermatitis (bumblefoot) lesions.

(a) What are likely to be the contributing factors causing these lesions?

(b) What treatment do you suggest?

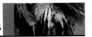

→ **28**

This foot of a northern goshawk *(Accipiter gentilis gentilis)* has a softish swelling that had been present on the foot for several years before examination. It remained the same size after its initial growth over the course of 2 to 3 months.
The owner wished it to be removed. How would you proceed?

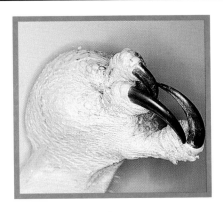

→ **29**

This newly acquired blue-fronted Amazon parrot *(Amazona aestiva)* presented with poor feathering around the fore part of the head and an abnormal upper beak.
(a) What kind of disease is likely to cause these clinical signs?
(b) How would you confirm your diagnosis?

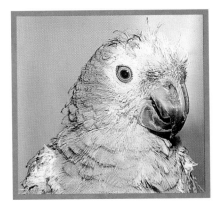

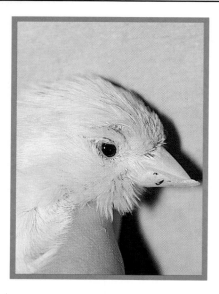

← 30

This young canary *(Serinus canaria)* has an abnormal lower beak. It is from a breeding flock in which other birds were showing the same signs.
(a) What is the possible etiology?
(b) What other clinical signs might you expect to see?

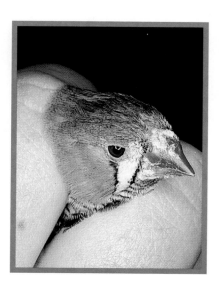

← 31

(a) What is the species of this bird?
(b) What is the likely cause of the lesion on its beak?
(c) How would you confirm your diagnosis?
(d) How would you treat the condition?

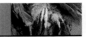

→ **32**
This raptor's rectrices are damaged.
(a) What are the possible causes?
(b) How is this condition prevented in hospitalized birds?

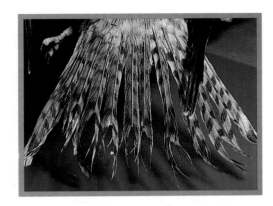

→ **33**
This parakeet was presented with persistent feather sheaths and with an associated parakeratosis. A simultaneous endoparasitic infection was also diagnosed. What is your diagnosis regarding these feather disorders?

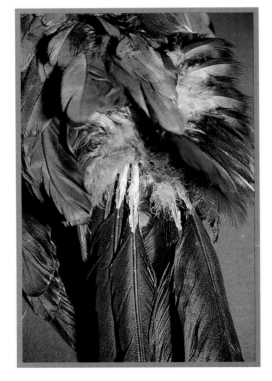

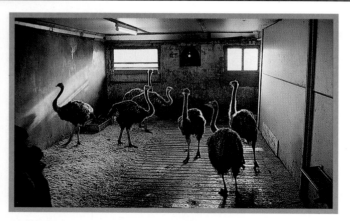

↑ 34
What are the main health hazards to these birds?

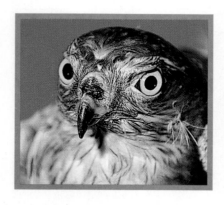

← 35
This is a sparrowhawk *(Accipiter nisus)*.
(a) What anatomic region of this bird has been traumatized?
(b) What underlying articulation may have been involved in this injury?
(c) What is the clinical significance of the underlying articulation?

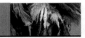

→ **36, 37**

These two budgerigars *(Melopsittacus undulatus)* and the accompanying postmortem illustration of another bird show the characteristics of a certain disease.

(a) What clinical signs are present?

(b) What is this disease?

(c) What other clinical signs might the bird on the left of the picture exhibit?

(d) What line of therapy would you adopt?

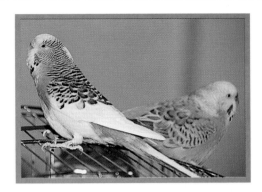

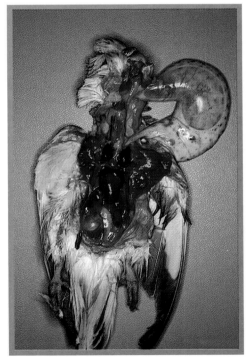

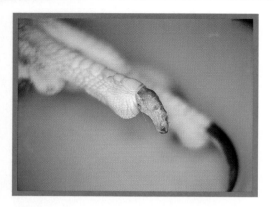

↑ **38**
This is the foot of a falcon presented with the
complete loss of the claw.
(a) What disorders of the claws could
account for this lesion?
(b) How would you treat this lesion?

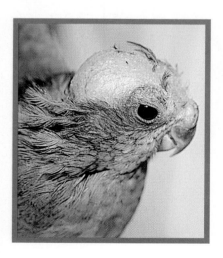

← **39**
This 6-year-old parrot presented
with a feather loss on the crown of
its head. Clinically, there were no
other findings.
(a) What is your tentative
diagnosis?
(b) How would you treat this
condition?

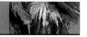

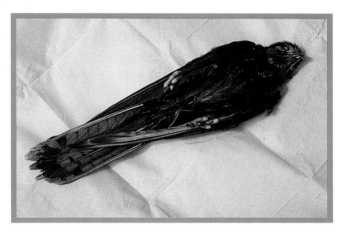

↑   **40**
This is a kestrel *(Falco tinnunculus)* that became severely oiled and comatose after being trapped in an oil sump at an oil refinery.
(a)   What do you know about oiled birds?
(b)   How should they be treated?

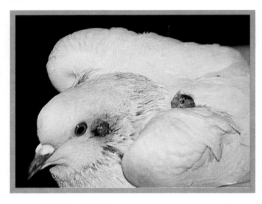

← **41, 42**
These illustrations demonstrate two clinical signs of the same disease. Fig. 41 shows numerous blood-filled granulomatous lesions on the skin. Fig. 42 shows papules of the oral mucous membrane.
(a) How would you diagnose this problem?
(b) What do you know about the possible disease?
(c) How would you treat this patient?

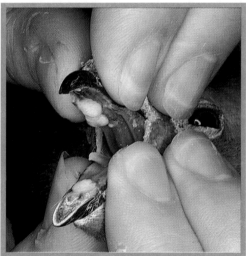

→ **43**

(a) Of what species is this bird a member?

(b) Where are its nares?

(c) What precautions should be taken when handling such birds?

(d) Are there any particular environment pollutants from which these birds are prone to injury?

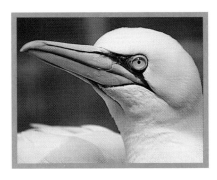

→ **44**

This Indian hill mynah *(Gracula religiosa)* presented with hanging wings and dyspnea.

(a) What do these signs indicate, especially if they are accompanied with marked abdominal swelling and ascites?

(b) What do you know of this condition commonly seen in mynah birds?

(c) How would you stabilize this obviously very ill bird?

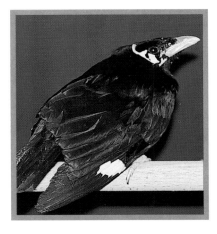

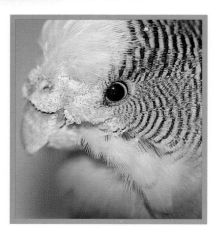

← **45**
This budgerigar *(Melopsittacus undulatus)* presented with crusty, honeycomb lesions around the beak, cere, and lores.
(a) What is your diagnosis?
(b) What other clinical signs might be seen?
(c) How can the condition be treated?

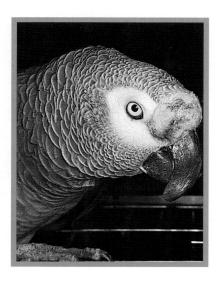

← **46**
This African grey parrot *(Psittacus erithacus)* presented with an abnormality of the cere and an associated scissor beak.
(a) What is your tentative diagnosis and how would you confirm this diagnosis?
(b) What is the prognosis?
(c) Would you consider corrective surgery to the beak?

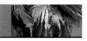

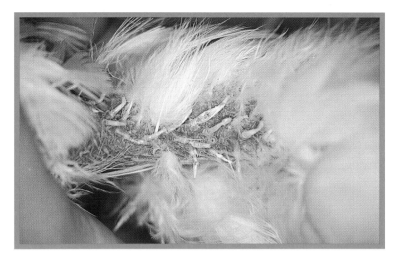

↑ → **47, 48**
What feather dystrophies do you see in these two illustrations?
(a) Of which disease is this characteristic?
(b) How would you confirm your diagnosis?

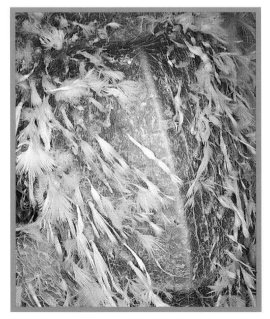

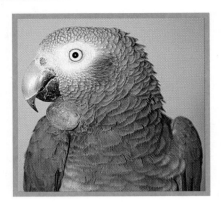

← 49

This grey parrot *(Psittacus erithacus)* has a submandibular swelling.
(a) What is the most likely etiology of this lesion?
(b) What are the possible differential diagnoses?
(c) What course of treatment would you suggest?

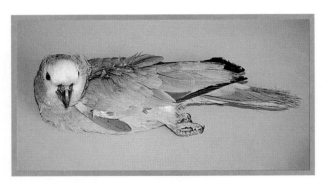

↑ 50

This blue-fronted Amazon parrot *(Amazona aestiva)* had been slightly "off color" for a few days; that is, its appetite was slightly reduced and it had not been as talkative as usual. Clinical examination revealed a slightly more prominent sternal keel bone. The feces were noted to contain very little urate. The owner found this bird on the bottom of its cage exhibiting what appeared to be paralysis of the legs.
(a) What is your tentative diagnosis
(b) What is your differential diagnosis?
(c) How would you proceed to confirm your diagnoses?

→ **55**

(a) Is the cere of this pigeon *(Columba livia)* normal?

(b) What is the sex of this bird?

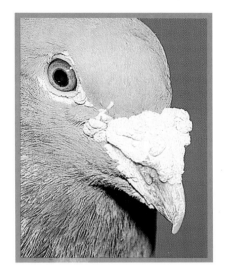

→ **56**

This raptor has an obvious problem with its feet and is having some difficulty perching.

(a) What is this condition called?

(b) What do you know about its etiology?

(c) What line of treatment would you adopt?

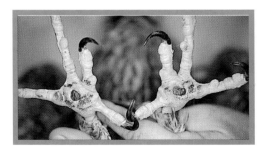

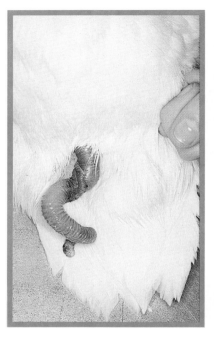

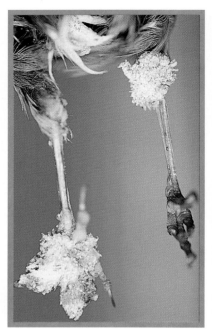

↑ 57
This is the pathologically extruded phallus of a domestic duck, which the bird is unable to retract.
(a) What do you notice about this organ?
(b) In what circumstances does this occur?
(c) Can anything be done to relieve this condition?

↑ 58
This picture shows the feet of a finch with papilloma-like lesions. What do you know about this disease?

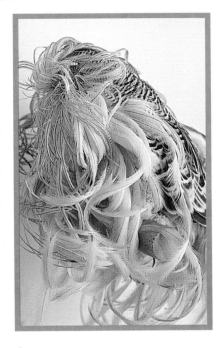

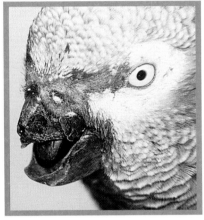

↑ 59

A feather dystrophy occasionally seen in British show budgerigars *(Melopsittacus undulatus)* is the so-called feather duster syndrome. (Courtesy Prof. Dr. Rautenfeld.) What do you know about this condition?

(a) What do you notice that is abnormal with the feathers?

(b) What is believed to be the etiology of this condition?

↑ 60

This severely injured African grey parrot *(Psittacus erithacus)* has suffered avulsion of most of the upper beak.

(a) Which underlying bone will have been affected?

(b) What is the prognosis for this bird?

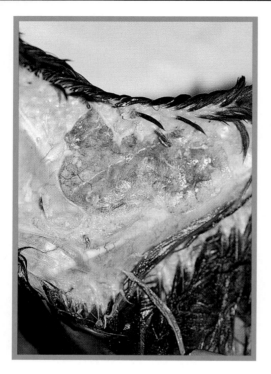

← 61

This is the propatagium of a Timneh grey parrot *(Psittacus erithacus timneh)*, which was presented with a skin disorder, after which it was treated by a veterinarian for several weeks using a locally applied ointment.

(a) What are the taxonomy and characteristics of this species of parrot?

(b) What type of environment does it normally inhabit?

(c) What do you know about iatrogenic feather disorders caused by the topical application of drugs to the skin and feathers?

→ 62

This mynah bird *(Gracula religiosa)* showed a feather loss and dermatitis in the submandibular region. There was no apparent pruritus or any other clinical signs. What is the likely etiology of this lesion?

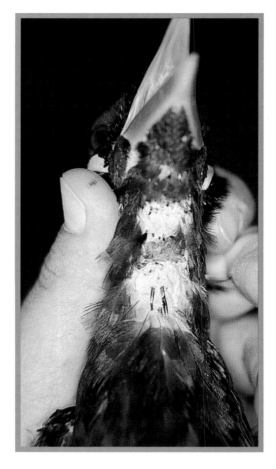

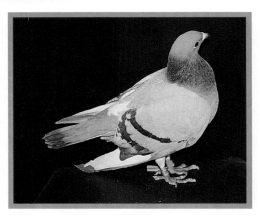

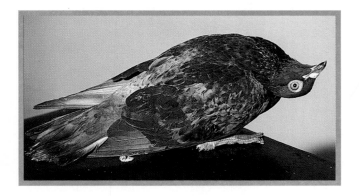

↑ 63, 64

Both of these pigeons *(Columba livia)* illustrate the clinical
signs of an infectious disease. Other clinical signs noted in
the birds in contact with that shown in Fig. 63 were
polydipsia, polyuria, and diarrhea.
(a) What is this disease?
(b) What other species of bird can it infect?
(c) If you were presented with only the pigeon illustrated
    in Fig. 63, what would be your differential diagnoses?

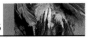

→ 65

These are the feet of a budgerigar *(Melopsittacus undulatus)*. The bird showed no other clinical signs.
(a) What is your provisional diagnosis
(b) How would you confirm this diagnosis?

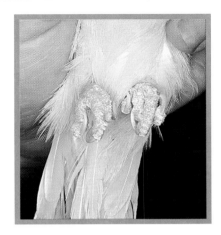

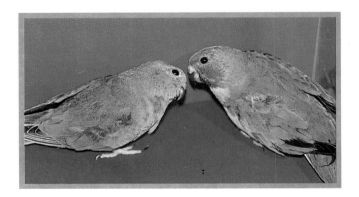

↑ 66

These two turquoise parrots *(Neophema pulchella)* are from an aviary in which some of the birds have developed diarrhea and central nervous system symptoms.
A salmonellosis was diagnosed.
(a) What differential diagnoses can you think of in the case demonstrated?
(b) How would you treat this flock?

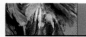

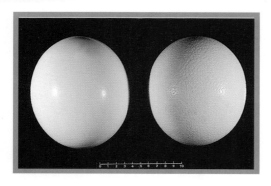

← 67

These two ostrich *(Struthio camelus)* eggs from an ostrich farm show differences in their surface texture. (Courtesy Dr. J. Baker.)

(a) Why aren't both eggs the same?

(b) What importance is this in the commercial production of ostrich chicks?

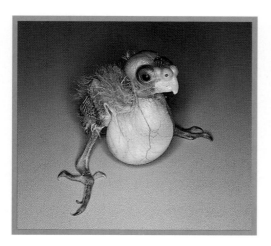

← 68

This picture shows a fledgling parrot with an overdistended crop.

(a) What are the causes of this condition?

(b) What type of therapy would you adopt?

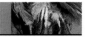

→ 69

This grey parrot *(Psittacus erithacus)* is a "feather picker."

(a) What do you know of this condition?
(b) What is the usual etiology?
(c) What are the characteristic clinical signs?
(d) How would you treat this bird?

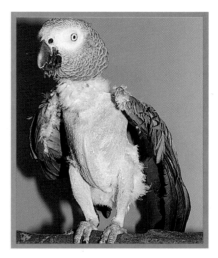

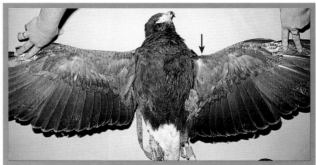

↑ 70

This raptor was said to fly abnormally, "like a butterfly." In the picture it has been deeply anaesthetized so that a thorough physical examination of the wings could be carried out. Both wings are held at full extension. The arrow indicates scar tissue formation. Radiography revealed no skeletal abnormality.

(a) Of what species is this bird?
(b) Can you deduce what has happened?
(c) Can anything be done to relieve this condition?

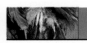

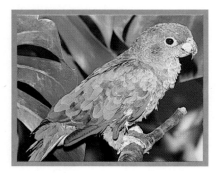

← 71

This blue-headed *Pionus* parrot *(Pionus menstruus)* shows a discoloration of the feathers from the normal green of the body plumage to partly black. The normal deep blue feathers on the head are faded, as is the red pigmentation of the base of both upper and lower beaks. Furthermore, there were signs of dyspnea. The referring veterinarian diagnosed a thyroid hyperplasia.

(a) What signs would you expect to see with thyroid disease?
(b) How would you confirm your diagnosis?
(c) Was the diagnosis of the referring veterinarian correct?

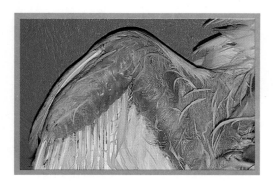

↑ 72

This is the wing of a young cockatoo presented with a marked swelling of the skin.

(a) What is your diagnosis of this condition?
(b) What is the possible etiology?
(c) In what other species do similar lesions occur?

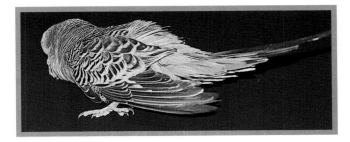

↑ 73
This acutely ill budgerigar *(Melopsittacus undulatus)*
presented with typical signs of shock.
(a) What clinical signs would you expect to see in a
    shocked bird?
(b) What emergency care routine is indicated?

→ 74
This illustration shows the
oropharynx of a feral
pigeon *(Columba livia),*
covered in caseous exudate
and with some bleeding.
(a) What do you know
    about the etiology of
    this lesion?
(b) What method of
    treatment would you
    adopt?

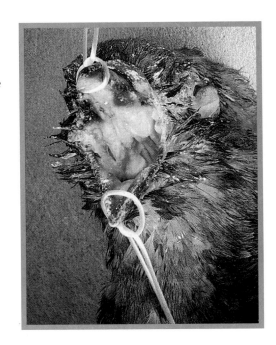

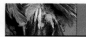
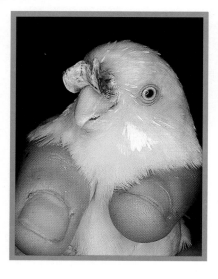

← 75
(a) What is the condition seen in this budgerigar *(Melopsittacus undulatus)*?
(b) Of what clinical significance is this condition?
(c) Can anything be done about it?

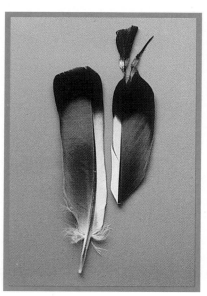

← 76
These dystrophic contour feathers, one of which is duplicated, are from a racing pigeon *(Columba livia)*. They developed after the owner had been treating the birds with an unknown drug. What do you know about iatrogenic feather disorders?

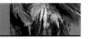
→ **77**

This female peach-faced love bird
(Agapornis roseicollis roseicollis) with
a history of chronic egg-laying over
the last several years was presented
with abnormal feathering and
weakness.

(a) What is your tentative
diagnosis?
(b) What kind of therapy would
you suggest?

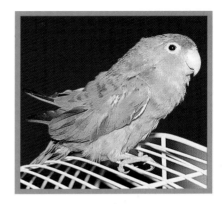

→ **78**

This is the foot of a
Philippine hanging parrot
*(Loriculus philippensis
bonapartei)* that was kept in
an outside aviary
throughout the year.

(a) To what cause do you
suspect the loss of the
claws is due?
(b) What advice would you
give the owner to
prevent this occurring
again?

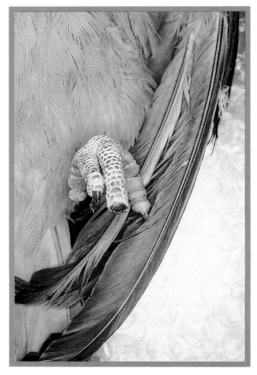

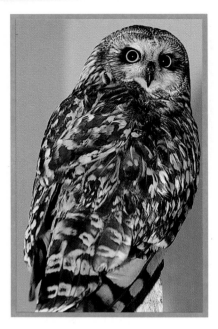

← 79

This wild short-eared owl *(Asia flammeus)* shows a dropped right wing and some signs of spoiled plumage in the region of the shoulder joint. What factors would you take into account before you would consider releasing this bird back into its wild habitat?

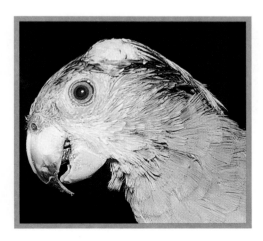

← 80

This blue-fronted Amazon parrot *(Amazona aestiva)* presented with a granulomatous mass on the head.

(a) What differential diagnosis would you consider?

(b) How could this be confirmed?

→ **81**

This cockatoo *(Eolophus roseicapillus)*, or galah, presented with bleeding and a longitudinal fracture of the lower beak. How would you treat this bird?

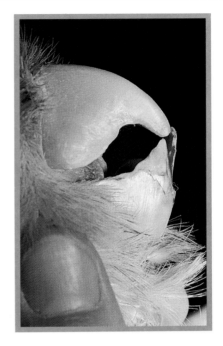

→ **82**

This canary has multiple feather defects.
(a) What is the possible etiology?
(b) In what breeds of canary is this most common
(c) In what other species of birds does this condition commonly occur?
(d) Is any treatment effective?

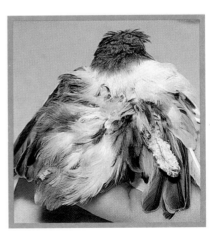

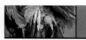

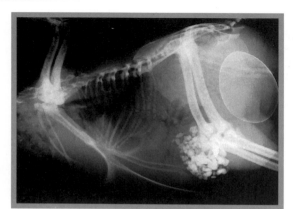

← 83
This is a laterolateral radiograph of the body of a fancy breed of chicken *(Gallus gallus)*. Comment on this radiograph.

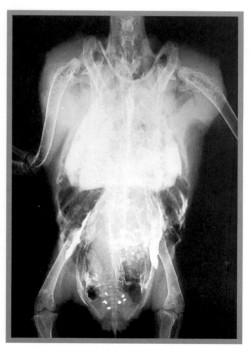

← 84
This is a ventrodorsal radiograph of an African grey parrot *(Psittacus erithacus)*. Comment on this radiograph.

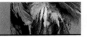

→ **85**

This is a greater barbet *(Megalaima virens)*, which is obviously favoring its left leg.
(a) What do you know of this type of bird and its life history?
(b) How would you investigate its lameness?

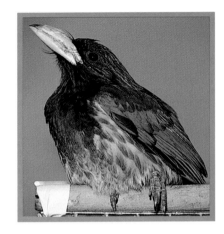

→ **86**

This aviary-kept lesser sulphur-crested cockatoo *(Cacatua sulphurea)* presented with central nervous system signs (torticollis) and diarrhea.
(a) What is your list of differential diagnoses?
(b) What would be your initial line of treatment to help to stabilize the patient before a definitive diagnosis was made?

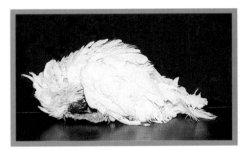

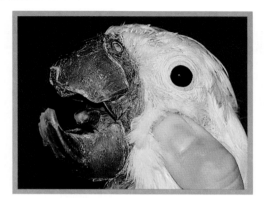

← 87

This cockatoo presented with a broken and ulcerated distal end of the upper beak and an overgrown mandibular beak. Physical examination of the bird revealed feather loss without pruritus, which apparently had been progressing for several months.
(a) What is your tentative diagnosis?
(b) What are the differential diagnoses?

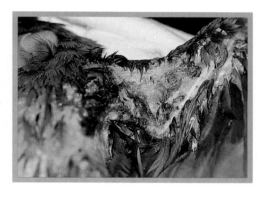

← 88

This lesion is situated on the propatagial membrane of a yellow-collared macaw *(Ara auricollis)*.
(a) What anatomic area of the bird is this?
(b) What is the apparent nature of this lesion?
(c) What micropathogens are likely to be involved?
(d) How would you arrive at a definitive diagnosis?

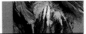

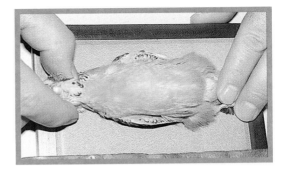

↑ 89

This budgerigar *(Melopsittacus undulatus)* is
being restrained for radiography.
(a) Comment on this procedure.
(b) What are other methods of restraining
birds for radiography?

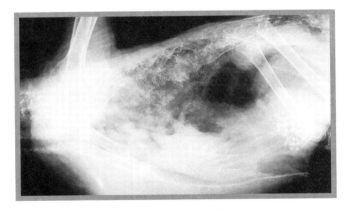

↑ 90

This is a laterolateral radiograph of a red-fronted macaw
(Ara rubrogenys) that was presented with dyspnea and was
apparently infertile. This male bird was kept with its partner
in an aviary for several years without contact with other
birds. What is your tentative diagnosis?

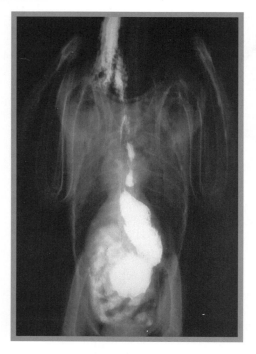

← 91
This is a ventrodorsal radiograph of the body of an African grey parrot *(Psittacus erithacus)* after the administration of a contrast medium.
(a) What are the common contrast media used for radiography in birds?
(b) What do you know about their application?

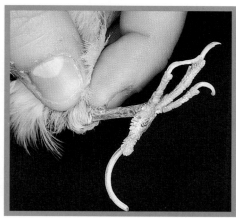

← 92
These are the feet of a canary *(Serinus canaria)*.
(a) What abnormalities can you see?
(b) What advice would you give the owner?

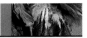

➜ **93**

This African grey parrot *(Psittacus erithacus)* is attempting to climb up the outside of its cage using its right leg and its beak. It is also fluttering its wings to assist in its ascent. This problem is of fairly acute onset. There were no other signs.

(a) From your observations, what are your tentative diagnoses?

(b) How would you confirm these?

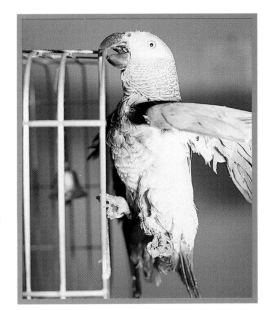

➜ **94**

This is the mouth of a galah cockatoo *(Eolophus roseicapillus)* showing the rima glottis brought into view by traction on the bird's tongue, which is held between the finger and thumb on the right side of the illustration.

(a) What abnormality do you see?

(b) What is the possible etiology?

(c) How can the diagnosis be confirmed?

(d) What method of treatment would you adopt?

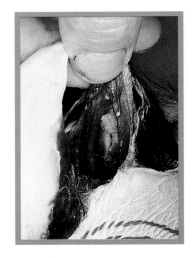

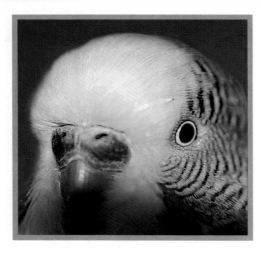

← 95
This 4-year-old budgerigar
(Melopsittacus undulatus)
presented with the normal
blue cere beginning to
change to brown. Further
clinical signs were cachexia,
dyspnea, and abdominal
swelling.
(a) What is your tentative
diagnosis?
(b) How would you confirm
this?

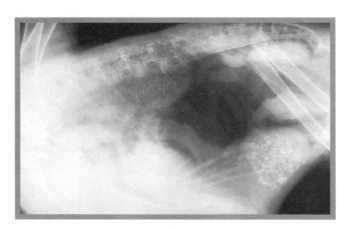

↑ 96
This is a laterolateral radiograph of an orange-winged
Amazon parrot *(Amazona amazonica)* that was brought to
the veterinarian for a routine check-up.
Comment on this radiograph.

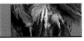

→ **97**

This African grey parrot *(Psittacus erithacus)* shows a blocked nostril.
(a) What is this lesion?
(b) What is your differential diagnosis?
(c) What can be done to relieve this condition?

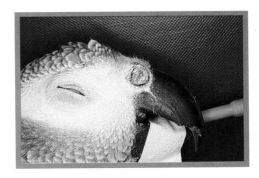

→ **98**

This red-lored Amazon parrot *(Amazona autumnalis)* was affected by a chronic glomerulonephritis eventually diagnosed at postmortem examination.
(a) What kinds of feather disorder are likely to be seen with renal diseases?
(b) What is your differential diagnoses in this case?
(c) What therapy would you suggest?

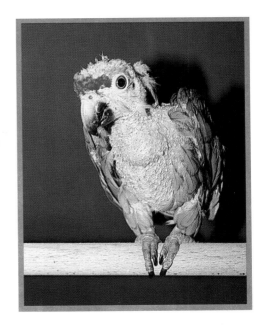

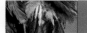

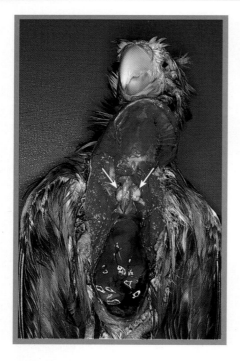

← **99**
This postmortem illustration of a parrot with the ribs cut and the sternum folded back cranially shows two abnormal structures as indicated by the arrows. These are signs typical of a certain disease.
(a) What is this disease?
(b) What do you know about this disease?

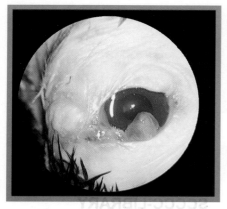

← **100**
This lovebird presented with eyelid lesions subsequent to a bite wound. (Courtesy Dr. Neumann.)
(a) Describe exactly the lesions you see.
(b) What are the possible causes of a prolapse of the nictitating membrane?
(c) How would you treat a prolapse?

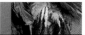

➜ **101**

This is the eye of an eagle owl *(Bubo bubo)* with a glaucoma. What do you know of glaucoma in birds? (Courtesy Dr. Neumann.)

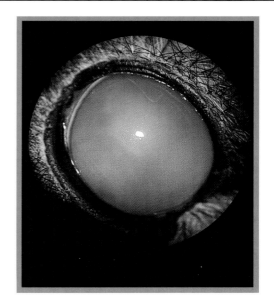

➜ **102**

This is a parasite, shown by microscopy, found at necropsy in a bird with respiratory distress.

(a)   In which species of birds is this parasite commonly found.

(b)   What do you know about this type of infestation?

(c)   How would you diagnose infestation?

(d)   What treatment can be used?

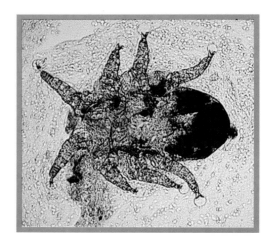

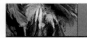
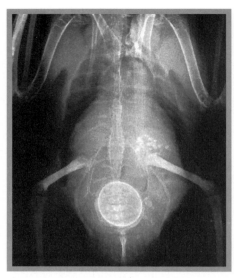

← 103
This is a ventrodorsal radiograph of a cockatiel *(Nymphicus hollandicus)*. Three weeks after laying 10 normally developed eggs the bird showed symptoms of egg binding.
(a) What signs would you expect to see with an egg-bound bird?
(b) Comment on this radiograph.
(c) What type of therapy would you propose?

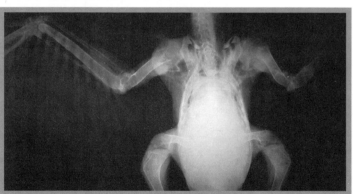

↑ 104
This is a dorsoventral radiograph of a wild, immature carrion crow *(Corvus corone)* found on the ground beneath its nest. It was being fed by the adult birds but appeared to the finder to be crippled.
(a) What observations can you make about this radiograph?
(b) From what condition is this bird suffering?

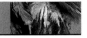

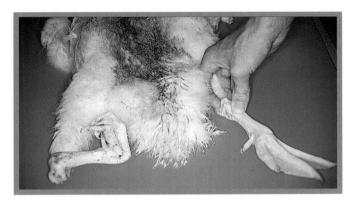

↑ **105**
This young domestic goose *(Anser anser)* shows luxation of
both tarsometatarsal joints.
(a) What is the presumed etiology of this condition?
(b) Which species of birds are similarly affected?
(c) What is your differential diagnosis?
(d) What therapy would you suggest?

→ **106**
These microorganisms
have been cultivated from
a swab taken from the
cloaca of a budgerigar
(Melopsittacus undulatus)
(Gram's stain).
(a) What are these
     microorganisms?
(b) What pathologic
     significance would
     you attribute to this
     finding?

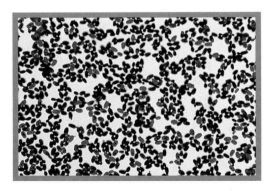

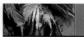

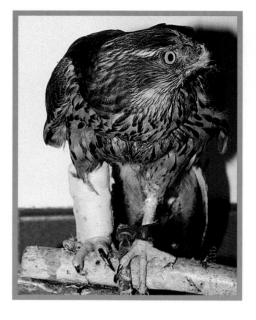

← 107

This Northern goshawk *(Accipiter gentilis gentilis)* has had a plaster cast placed on its leg to stabilize a fracture of the tibiotarsus. Comment on this procedure and what you notice in the picture.

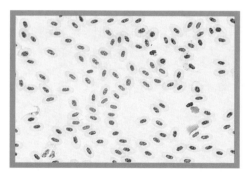

← 108

This blood smear was obtained from a mynah bird *(Gracula religiosa)*. Two hematozoan parasites can be seen in this sample (magnification ×500).

(a) What are the parasites seen?

(b) What do you know of trypanosomes in birds in general, and of what clinical significance are they?

(c) What do you know of avian malarial parasites, and of what clinical significance are they?

→ **109**

This blue-fronted Amazon parrot *(Amazona aestiva)* presented with chemosis of the conjunctiva, uveitis, and secondary cataract. (Courtesy Dr. Neumann.)
(a) Explain the term chemosis.
(b) What kind of causal agent would you suspect?

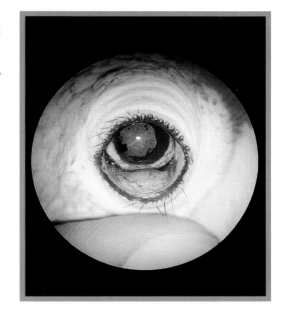

→ **110**

Defects of the cornea after traumatic insults (e.g., bites) are commonly seen, such as in this common kestrel *(Falco tinnunculus)*. In this bird, fluorescein has been applied to highlight the defect. (Courtesy Dr. Neumann.)
(a) Comment on this technique and on the prognosis for this condition.
(b) What treatment would you use?
(c) What are the possible complications of this lesion?

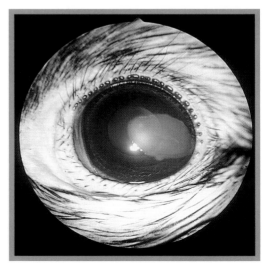

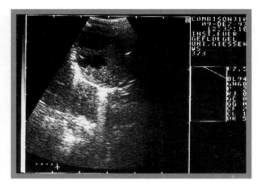

← 111

This is an ultrasonographic picture of the kidney of a budgerigar *(Melopsittacus undulatus)* suffering from paresis of the legs. What comments do you have on this picture?

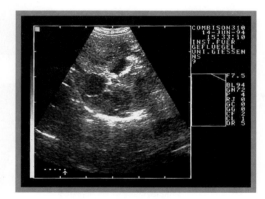

← 112

A female cockatiel *(Nymphicus hollandicus)* is presented with abdominal distention, dyspnea, and problems passing feces. Radiography showed a diffuse shadow in the abdominal region, a craniodorsal displacement of the gizzard, and the formation of medullary bone. Ultrasonography of the genital tract shows the picture illustrated. What can you see and how would you interpret these findings?

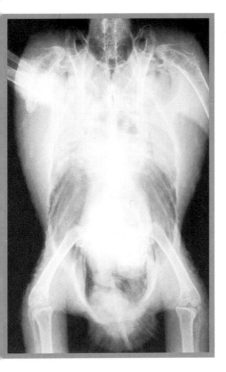

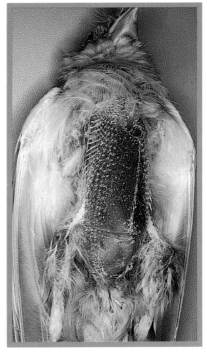

↑ **113**
This is a ventrodorsal radiograph of
the body of an African grey parrot
(Psittacus erithacus). The bird was
presented with diarrhea, dyspnea,
and apathy. The owner reported
that, after trauma 5 days previously,
the bird was unable to fly. Based on
the radiograph, what is your
diagnosis?

↑ **114**
This is the body of a captive-bred
greenfinch *(Carduelis chloris)* that
was plucked before autopsy. The
owner lost several of these birds of
various ages over the course of
several weeks. The birds continued
to feed and, although only slightly
depressed, behaved normally. The
only signs observed by the owner
were that they were "going light,"
that is, slowly losing weight. List
your differential diagnoses in order
of the most likely cause and briefly
give the reasons for your choices.

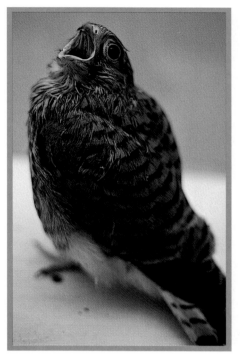

← 115

This young kestrel *(Falco tinnunculus)* was taken from the wild and reared artificially.
(a) What does the behavior it is exhibiting indicate?
(b) How difficult will it be to rehabilitate this bird back into its natural wild habitat?

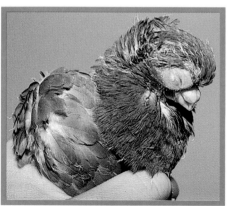

← 116

This pigeon showed bilateral periocular swelling. What etiology would you suspect for this condition?

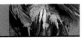

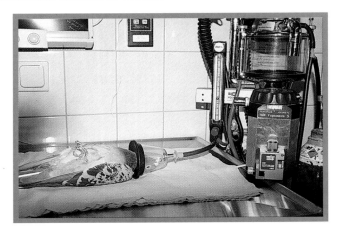

→ **117**

This pigeon is under inhalant anesthesia. What inhalant anesthetics can be used for birds?

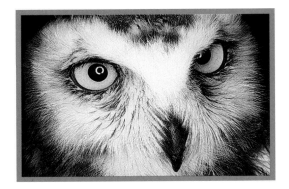

↑ **118**

(a) What do you know about the pupil of the avian eye.
(b) What do you know about the lens?

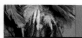

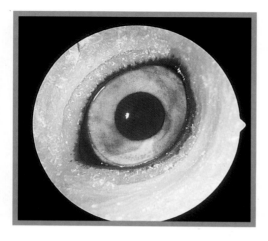

← **119**
(a) What do you know about the physiologic color of the avian iris?
(b) When is discoloration likely to occur?

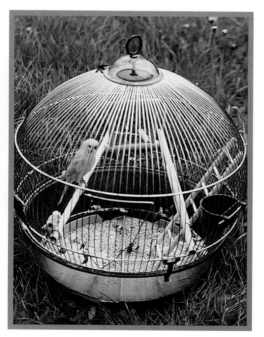

← **120**
What advice would you give to the owner about improving the welfare of this small caged bird?

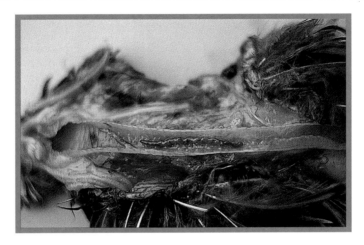

↑ 121

This trachea of a pheasant contains several parasites.
(a) What are these parasites?
(b) Which species of birds can they infect?
(c) Describe the life cycle of the parasite and the symptoms these parasites cause in birds.

→ 122

These are the castings of a common buzzard *(Buteo buteo)*.
(a) What can be noted about these castings?
(b) Are they normal?

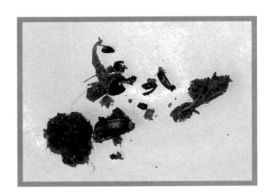

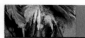

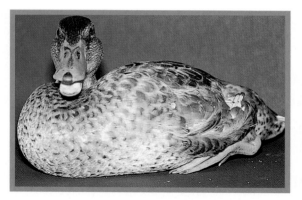

← 123
This duck was observed to be mouth-breathing and was presented with a sudden onset of severe dyspnea and rales in the upper respiratory tract. What initial treatment would you suggest?

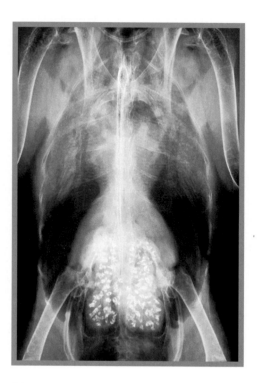

← 124
This dorsoventral radiograph of an African gray parrot *(Psittacus erithacus)* shows radiodense structures within the kidneys.
(a) What are these radiodense structures?
(b) What may their presence suggest?

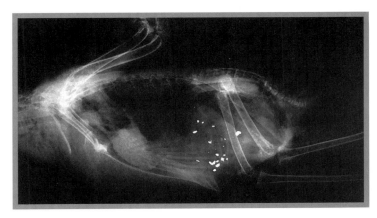

↑ 125
(a) What is the most obvious abnormality shown in this laterolateral radiograph of a psittacine bird?
(b) This bird exhibited sudden signs of weakness, ataxia, and a tendency to convulsion. What is your diagnosis?
(c) What are your suggestions for therapy?

→ 126
The owner of this African gray parrot *(Psittacus erithacus)* reports that a "tumor" has been growing on the head of this bird during the last few weeks. He now wants to know about the importance of this growth.

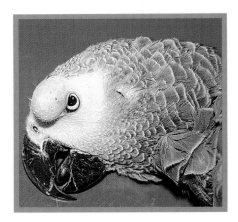

(a) For which condition is this localization typical?
(b) What would be your first question to the owner?
(c) How would you treat this patient?
(d) What other pathologies might be coexistent?

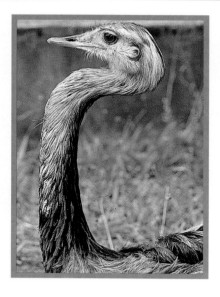

← **127**

This common, or greater, rhea *(Rhea americana)* has a cervical vertebral dislocation. What is the usual cause for this lesion in ratites?

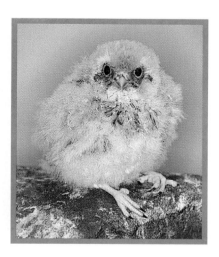

← **128**

This healthy wild fledgling raptor has been presented for advice regarding rearing.
(a) Approximately how old is this chick?
(b) What general advice would you give the person rearing the chick?
(c) What advice would you give if the fledgling is to be reared so that it can be rehabilitated back into the wild?
(d) What advice would you give if it were to be reared so that it could be used for falconry?

→ **129**

This budgerigar *(Melopsittacus undulatus)* presented with a continually moist area dampening the plumage over the rostral area of the sternum. Also, some seed was noticed sticking to the area. The owner reported the signs were of acute onset and otherwise the bird appeared to be quite normal.

(a) What is your tentative diagnosis?

(b) How would you confirm this?

(c) How would you resolve the problem?

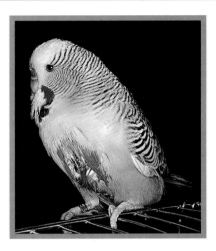

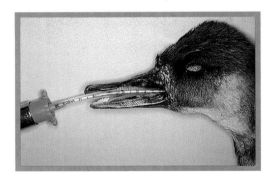

↑ **130**

This intubated duck has lost most of the lateral edge of its upper beak through some unknown traumatic incident.

(a) Can anything be done to resolve this condition?

(b) What is the long-term prognosis for this bird?

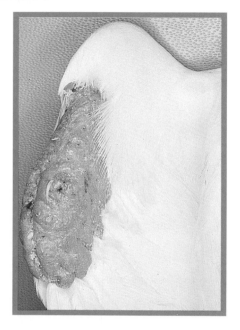

← 131
This lesion occurred over the metacarpophalangeal area of the wing of a cockatiel *(Nymphicus hollandicus)*.
(a) Describe the lesion.
(b) How would you confirm your diagnosis?
(c) How would you treat the problem?

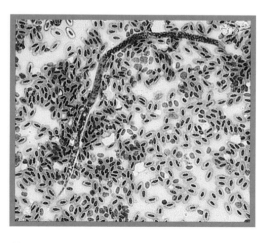

← 132
(a) What is the filiform structure visible in this avian blood?
(b) What pathologic importance would you attribute to this finding?
(Courtesy Dr. Balks.)

→ 133
A chicken is presented with severe lesions of the legs.
(a) What is your diagnosis?
(b) In which species and type of husbandry is this condition commonly seen?
(c) What is your suggested therapy?

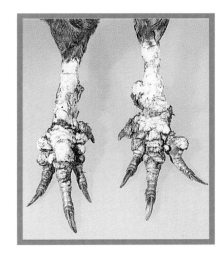

→ 134
This male blackbird *(Turdus merula)* flew into a windowpane. It is sitting on its hocks and tail feathers, showing paralysis of both legs. Apart from this, the bird seems to be alert, and radiographic examination did not reveal any pathologic condition.
(a) What is your comment on this disorder?
(b) What action would you take?

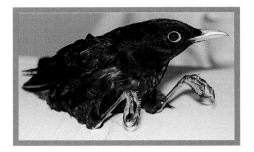

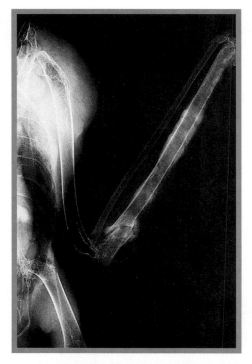

← 135

(a) What pathologic alteration does this radiograph of the wing of a common buzzard *(Buteo buteo)* show?

(b) How would you treat such a patient?

↓ 136

What is your comment on this necropsy specimen of a common starling *(Sturnus vulgaris)*?

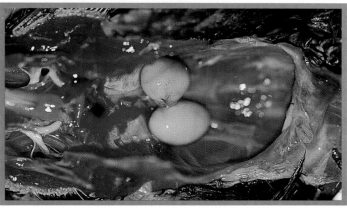

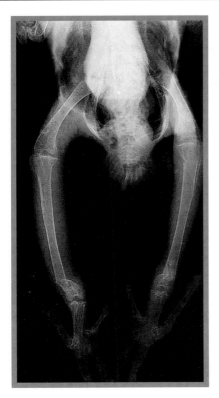

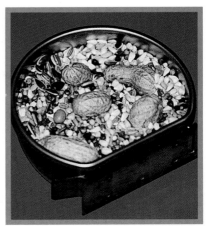

← 137, A, ↑ B
This illustration shows the radiograph of an African gray parrot *(Psittacus erithacus)* **(A)** and the sole diet **(B)** of this bird. What are your observations on this case?

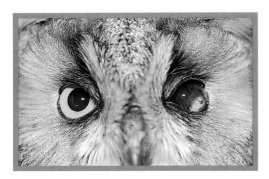

← 138
This great horned owl *(Bubo virginianus)* presented with a hyphema. What are your comments on this condition regarding etiology, prognosis, and treatment?

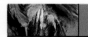

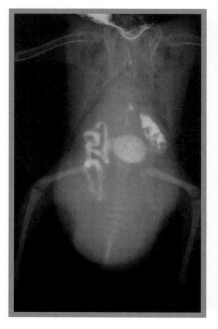 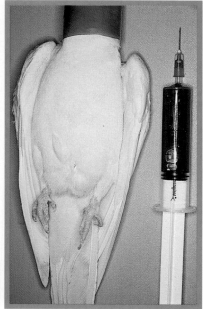

↑   **139, A, B**

A, Radiograph of a cockatiel *(Nymphicus hollandicus)* after barium positive-contrast media has been administered. **B,** The same cockatiel in dorsal recumbency under general anesthesia after 10 ml of dark brown colored fluid has been withdrawn via peritoneal paracentesis.

(a) From what you can see, what is your provisional diagnosis?

(b) How would you continue to treat this condition?

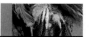
→ 140

This female blue-fronted Amazon parrot *(Amazona aestiva)* was presented with an abnormal mass in the caudal abdominal region. The bird was apathetic and had problems defecating. The bird's weight was 980 g.

(a) What is your tentative diagnosis?

(b) What kind of therapy would you suggest?

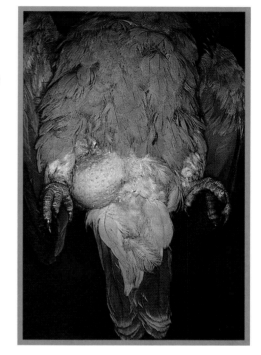

→ 141

This sample of droppings was passed by an African gray parrot *(Psittacus erithacus)* that weighed 300 g. The bird's appetite was normal and there were no other signs. The owner had fed the bird a good mixed diet including fruit and fresh vegetables, among which was some beetroot.

(a) What observations can you make?

(b) What are your differential diagnoses and how would you confirm these?

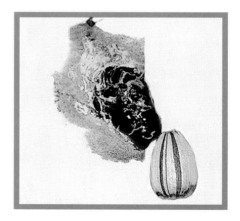

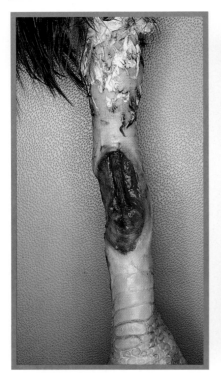

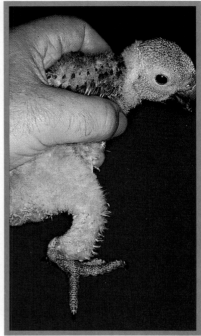

↑ **142**

This illustration shows deep ulceration of rostal surface of the tarsometatarsus of a Harris' hawk *(Parabuteo unicinctus)* as a result of a constricting identification closed band.

(a) What is the blackened strip of tissue running down the center of this lesion?

(b) What routine would you follow to help resolve this problem?

↑ **143**

This fledgling African gray parrot *(Psittacus erithacus)* is one of a clutch of three young parrots. It is unable to stand properly. From what you can see, what is your provisional diagnosis?

→ **144**

This budgerigar
(Melopsittacus undulatus)
presented with a pendulous
swelling of its abdomen.
(a) What is your diagnosis?
(b) What is the etiology of
the condition?
(c) How would you proceed
with treatment?

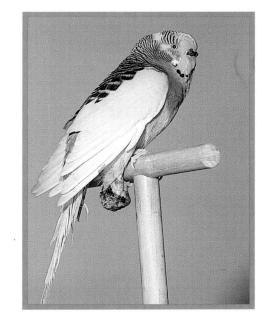

→ **145**

This is a traumatized Northern
goshawk *(Accipiter gentilis
gentilis)*.
(a) What pathologic signs
can be seen in this bird?
(b) Is this an old or a young
individual?
(c) What tests are indicated?

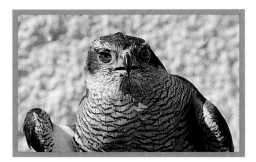

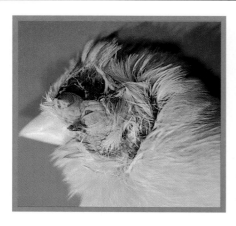

← **146**

This canary *(Serinus canaria)* was presented with severe lesions on its head. A tentative diagnosis of infection with pox virus was made.

(a) What are the various manifestations of canary pox?

(b) What symptoms would you expect to see in other birds of this group?

(c) How would you confirm your tentative diagnosis of pox virus infection?

(d) Apart from canaries the owner keeps racing pigeons and is worried about cross infection. What advice would you give?

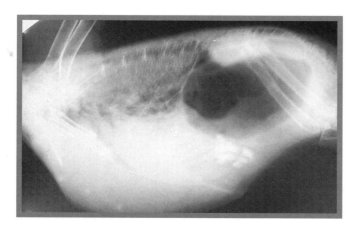

↑ **147**

A gray parrot *(Psittacus erithacus)* was presented with dyspnea. What phenomenon can you see in this radiograph and what is it caused by?

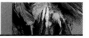

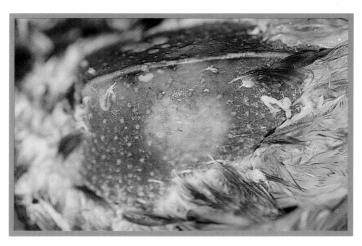

↑ **148**

A gray parrot *(Psittacus erithacus)* was presented with a swollen and necrotic lesion in its breast muscle. What are the likely causes?

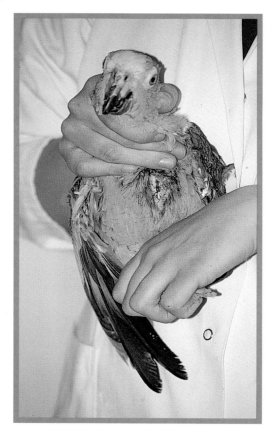

← 149
(a) What is wrong with this method of restraint?
(b) What improvements would you suggest?

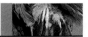

➔ **150**
What abnormalities are seen in this peripheral blood smear of a common buzzard *(Buteo buteo)?* (Giemsa; ×1000.) (Courtesy Dr. Balks.)
(a) What might be the underlying cause?
(b) How would you confirm your diagnosis?

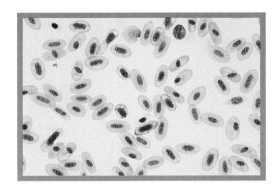

➔ **151**
This is a ventrodorsal radiograph of a budgerigar *(Melopsittacus undulatus).* Comment on the changes you see in this radiograph and on their clinical significance.

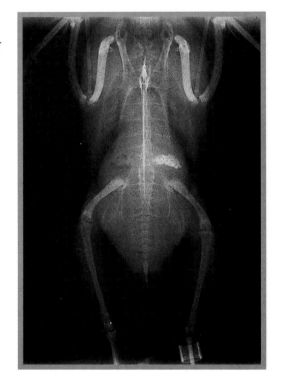

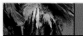

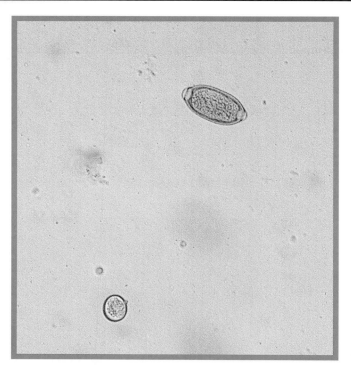

↑ 152
A client complains about the poor health of his flock of
racing pigeons. A few birds have died, and some have
diarrhea and are lethargic. Fecal examination reveals a few
coccidial oocysts and some eggs of *Capillaria* spp.
(a) What conclusions would you draw from these
observations?
(b) What measures would you initiate?

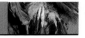

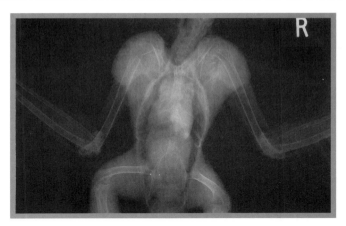

↑ 153

This is a dorsoventral radiograph of a tawny owl *(Strix aluco)* the owner had acquired some time previously. The client reported that the bird had been unable to fly since fledging and inquired if anything could be done to enable it to fly.

(a) What abnormalities do you see?

(b) Can anything be done to resolve this condition?

↑ **154**

This illustration made of a parrot at postmortem examination shows a duodenum packed with nematodes.

(a) What type of nematodes are these most likely to be?

(b) How could this bird have become infected?

(c) What would be the most likely antemortem clinical signs?

(d) What treatment would you prescribe?

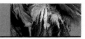

→ 155

(a) What species of bird is shown in this illustration?
(b) What is its natural prey?
(c) How would you feed such a bird if you had to hospitalize it?

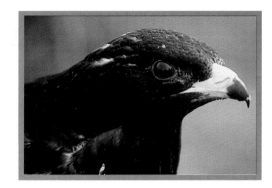

→ 156

This radiograph is of a European kestrel *(Falco tinnunculus)*. When found, it was unable to fly properly. The finder reported that no fractures were palpable. Although the bird ate normally, it lost weight and showed no improvement in ability to fly. Examination of this bird did not reveal any visible or palpable abnormalities of the locomotor system.

(a) What might be the causative disease?
(b) How would you confirm your tentative diagnosis?
(c) What treatment would you suggest?

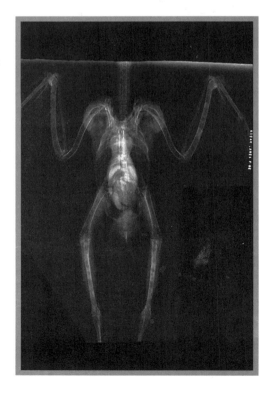

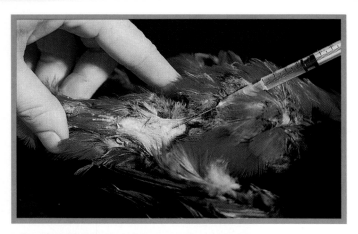

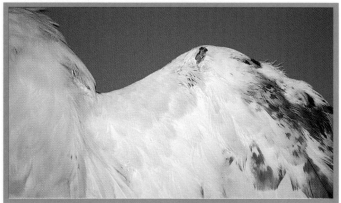

↑ 157, A, B

A and **B** demonstrate two injection techniques suitable for birds.

(a) What procedures are being performed? State the methods used and comment on the precautions the operator should take.

(b) In what circumstances would these two different methods of injection be used and what are their advantages compared with other injection techniques?

→ **158**

This is an ophthalmoscopic view of the avian fundus. (Courtesy Dr. Neumann.)

(a) Comment on the color of these structures.

(b) What do you know about the anatomy and physiology of the avian fundus?

(c) What type of pathologic changes may take place and what may be their etiology?

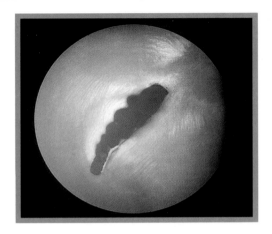

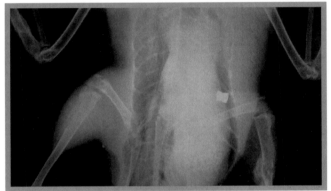

↑ **159**

This is the dorsoventral radiographic projection of a wild mallard duck *(Anas platyrhynchos)* presented by a wildlife rehabilitator. The bird was lame and had a wound on its left leg. The wildlife rehabilitator did not want the bird euthanized.

(a) What can you deduce from this radiograph?

(b) If asked that the duck's condition be restored to as near normal as possible so that the bird could be released, how would you proceed?

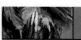
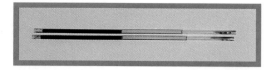

↑ 160

This illustration shows two microhematocrit capillary tubes containing a peripheral blood sample after centrifugation. (Courtesy Dr. Balks.)

(a) What information can be obtained from these tubes?

(b) Comment on plasma color, volume, and protein content.

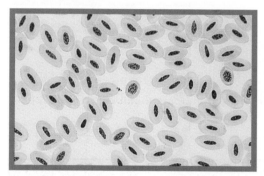

↑ 161

This illustration demonstrates a blood smear from a white stork *(Ciconia ciconia).* (Giemsa stain.) (Courtesy Dr. Balks.)

(a) What kind of cells are in the center and at the 3 o'clock position?

(b) What kinds of erythroid cells are found in the smears of avian peripheral blood?

(c) What do you know about the development of these cells, their reactions to different stains, and their classification?

(d) What is the significance of the finding in the particular case illustrated?

→ **162**

These are fledgling
finches.
(a) Do you notice
anything abnormal
about their general
attitude?
(b) What is the likely
cause of this
condition?

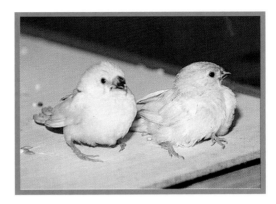

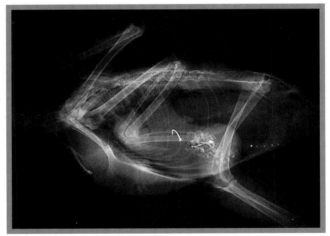

↑ **163**

This is the laterolateral radiograph of a moorhen (*Gallinula
chlorpus*) that was presented with a length of
monofilament nylon fishing line protruding from its
mouth. Although this radiograph is sufficient for diagnosis
in this case, the clarity would have been better had the
image of one wing not been superimposed on the body.
Although the diagnosis is obvious, what decision should
be made regarding this bird?

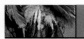

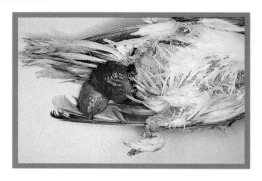

← 164

This hybrid lovebird (*Agapornis* spp.) presented with a cloacal prolapse.
(a) Which organs could possibly be involved in this prolapse?
(b) What clinical history and signs would guide you in making a diagnosis?
(c) How would you proceed therapeutically in resolving this case?

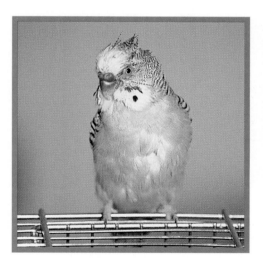

← 165

This budgerigar (*Melopsittacus undulatus*) presented with matted feathering around the paraorbital areas and over the back of the head. The bird was quite bright in demeanor.
(a) What do these signs indicate?
(b) How would you confirm your diagnosis?

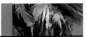

→ **166**

This Fischer's lovebird *(Agapornis fischeri)* was presented with an abnormal unilateral proptosis subsequent to a bite by a cage mate.
(a) What is the probable cause of this condition?
(b) What are your differential diagnoses?
(c) What is the prognosis for the case illustrated?

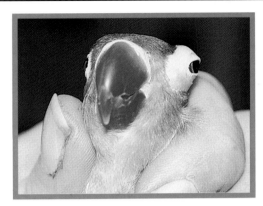

→ **167**

This liver impression smear was taken from an African gray parrot *(Psittacus erithacus).* (Ziehl-Neelsen; ×200.)
(a) Identify the structure in the centre of the image.
(b) Does this have any pathologic significance in this species?
(c) What is the comparative pathogenicity in other species of birds?

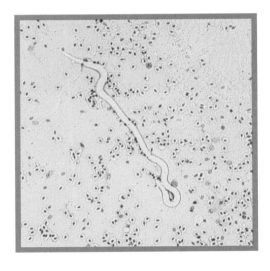

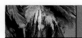

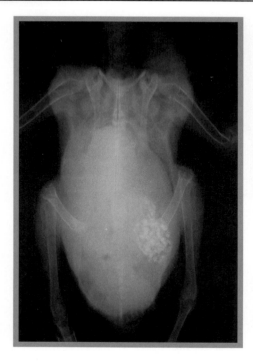

← **168**
This is the ventrodorsal radiograph of a female racing pigeon *(Columba livia)*. Its weight was 480 g, and it had difficulty flying. It was dyspneic. The bird was anesthetized for radiography using an injection into the pectoral muscle of ketamine and xylazine. Recovery was uneventful. What information can you gain from this radiograph?

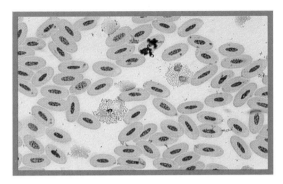

↑ **169**

This is a blood smear of a white stork *(Ciconia ciconia)*. (Pappenheim's stain; ×1000.)

Two types of granulocytic cells are shown in this picture. (Courtesy Dr. Balks.)

(a) Which types of granulocytic cells are shown?

(b) Where are they situated?

(c) What are the basic criteria for the differentiation of these two kinds of granulocyte?

(d) What influence do faulty staining technique and species of bird have on the staining characteristics of the granulocytes?

(e) What might be the cause or causes for degranulation?

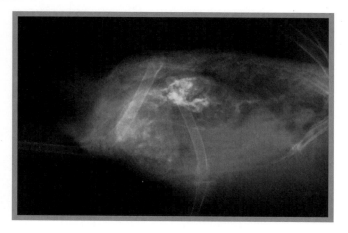

↑ 170

This is the laterolateral radiograph of a Timneh gray parrot *(Psittacus erithacus timneh)*. A diluted solution of barium contrast media had been administered 30 minutes before radiography. This bird was thin, had intermittent attacks of vomiting, and was showing signs of undigested seed in the droppings during the previous few months. The bird was presented in a collapsed condition.

(a) What is your diagnosis?

(b) Which species does this condition affect and what is its etiology?

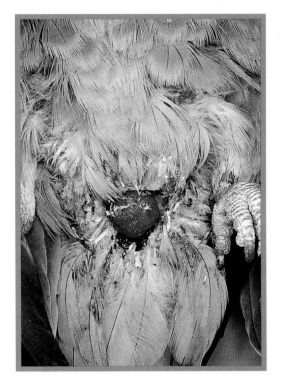

↑   **171**

This surgically sexed male Amazon parrot (*Amazona* spp.) has a cloacal prolapse. The owner had not noticed the prolapse and only reported blood in the droppings.

(a)   What are your differential diagnoses and what is the most likely etiology?

(b)   What investigations should you perform?

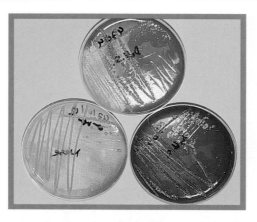

← 172

This illustration shows three bacterial agar plates culturing a fecal sample of a psittacine bird. In a psittacine bird, what general rules should you consider for a routine bacteriologic examination before reaching a decision about the primary pathogen?

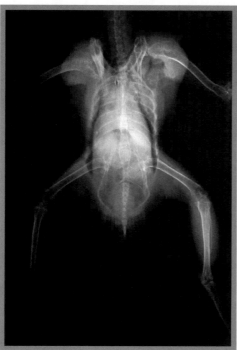

← 173

This is the ventrodorsal radiograph of a wild kestrel *(Falco tinnunculus)*. At presentation the bird was unable to fly and was rather thin.

(a) What is your diagnosis?
(b) How long do you think the bird has been injured?
(c) What are the prospects for the resolution of this condition?
(d) How would you achieve this?

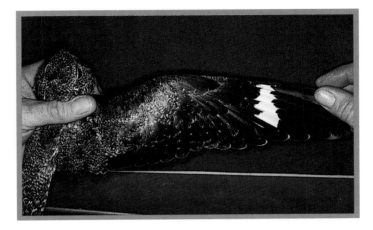

↑　**174**

This wild bird was presented by a municipal park warden, to whom it had been taken after being found in a private home garden on the west coast of England during the autumn. The bird was very thin but otherwise apparently normal.

(a)　Can you give the taxon of this bird?
(b)　Where is its normal range?
(c)　Can you account for the bird having been found in that particular location?
(d)　How would you deal with this case? Suggest methods of feeding and returning the bird to the wild.

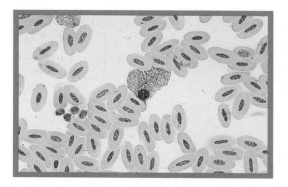

↑ **175**

This blood smear is from a white stork *(Ciconia ciconia).* (Pappenheim's stain; ×1000.) (Photograph courtesy of Dr. Balks.)

(a) In the centre of the picture is an inverted triangular group of three white blood cells. What cell is shown at the base (i.e., between and below) of the two heterophilic granulocytes?

(b) Is there a pathologic significance to the presence of this cell?

(c) Are these types of cells more commonly seen in some groups of birds?

(d) A group of four cells are also shown to the left and below the above cellular group. What are these cells, and what is their particular significance?

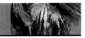

→ 176

This illustration shows the ventral aspect of a mature mutant (Lutino) Patagonian conure *(Cyanoliseus patagonus).* This bird was presented because of maldirected toes, which had been like this since hatching. The owner wished this condition to be corrected.

(a) What do you notice abnormal about these feet? What do you know about the normal detailed anatomy of psittacine birds' feet?

(b) Can you suggest what might be the problem and how can it be resolved?

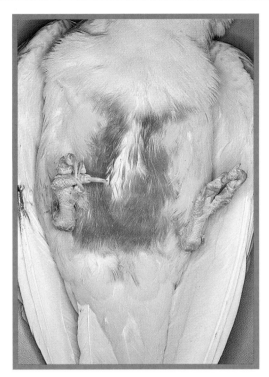

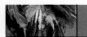

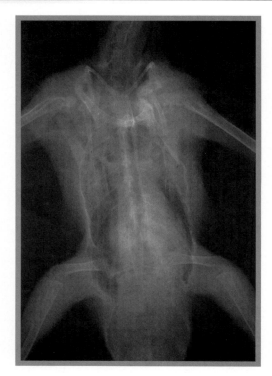

← **177**

This radiograph is the ventrodorsal projection of a black-headed gull *(Larus ridibundus)*. The bird was presented by a wildlife rehabilitator who had cared for the bird for 2 to 3 weeks as it convalesced from an injury.
(a) What abnormality can you see?
(b) What is the chance of the bird flying again?
(c) The bird was found in the center of England, far from the sea. Is this normal for this species?

→ 178

This anesthetized budgerigar *(Melopsittacus undulatus)* was presented with a lesion just below the left eye.
(a) Do you think this lesion is important?
(b) How would you advise the owner?

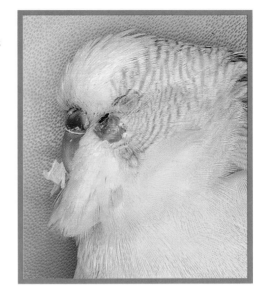

→ 179

This yellow-cheeked Amazon parrot *(Amazona xanthops)* presented with an obviously diseased eye and a dilated unresponsive pupil. What is your diagnosis? Discuss the clinical signs seen in this picture.

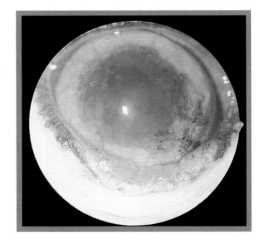

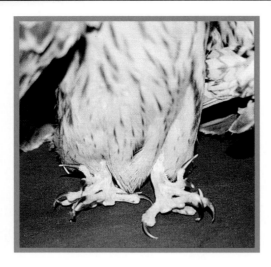

← 180

(a) What disorder can be seen in this young European kestrel *(Falco tinnunculus)?*

(b) What do you know about the etiology of these kinds of defects in birds?

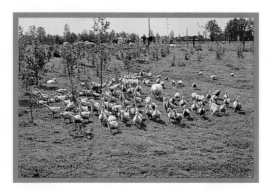

← 181

Discuss the principle methods of administering drugs orally to both single individuals and birds kept in flocks. What are the advantages and disadvantages of these various methods?

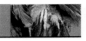

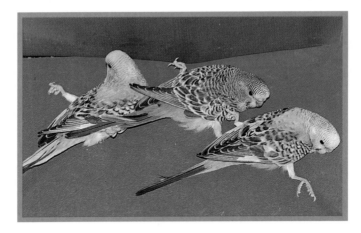

↑ **182**

(a) What do you notice wrong with these budgerigars *(Melopsittacus undulatus)?* What is the condition called and what is its cause?

(b) How can it be treated?

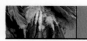

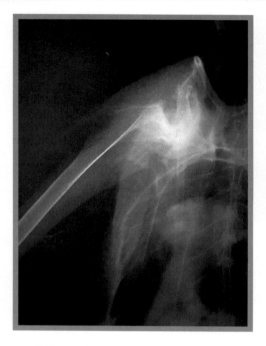

← 183

This radiograph is of the shoulder and part of the thorax of an immature herring gull *(Larus argentatus)*. This bird was a wildlife casualty with an injured wing, which the finder kept strapped for several weeks. When the bird was eventually presented to a veterinarian for advice it was unable to fly.

(a) What do you think has happened?
(b) How should the bird have been treated?

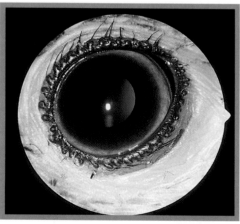

← 184

(a) Discuss the musculature and innervation of the avian pupil.
(b) What do you know about the physiologic color of the iris? When may discoloration occur?
(c) What do you know about the avian lens?

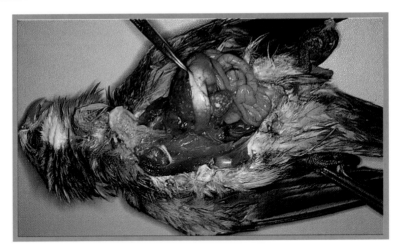

↑   **185**

This illustration of a superb parrot *(Polytelis swainsonii)* was made at postmortem examination. The artery forceps *(on the right of the illustration)* are attached to the duodenum, which has been pulled to the side so that both the liver and spleen are visible. The breeder reported intermittent sudden deaths during the latter part of the year in birds he kept in an outside aviary.

(a)   What pathology do you see?
(b)   What are your differential diagnoses?
(c)   How would you investigate this problem?
(d)   What advice would you give the owner?

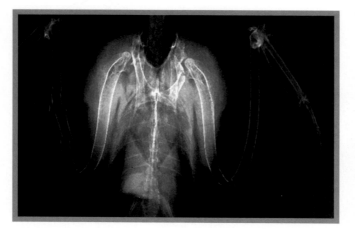

↑ **186**

This ventrodorsal radiograph is of a European sparrow-hawk *(Accipiter nisus)* that was presented with a dropped wing.
(a) What is your diagnosis?
(b) What therapy would you suggest and what precautions would you take?

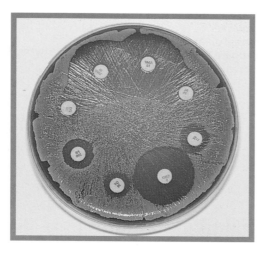

← **187**
What factors must be considered concerning antibiotic therapy if a sensitivity test for an antibiogram has been performed?

→ **188**

In this photomicrograph, a heterophilic granulocyte and mononuclear cell *(on the right)* are shown.
(a) Identify and in detail describe this type of cell.
(b) What disease processes are associated with the presence of these cells?

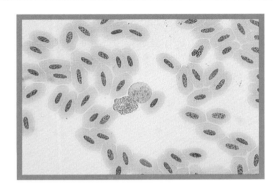

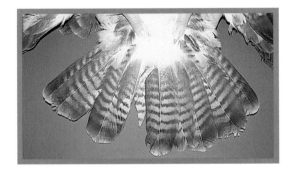

↑ **189**

This raptor, a goshawk *(Accipiter gentilis gentilis)*, has a broken tail feather.
(a) Does this damage have a marked influence on flight capability?
(b) What are the possibilities of the bird regaining normal plumage?
(c) Can damaged plumage be artificially repaired?

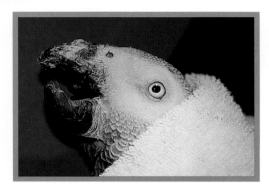

← **190**
This African gray parrot
(Psittacus erithacus) has a
necrotic lesion of the beak.
(a) What may be the
cause of this lesion?
(b) How would you
treat it?

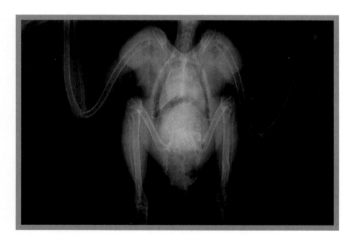

↑ **191**
This is the ventrodorsal radiograph of a wild tawny owl
(Strix aluco) that was involved in a traffic accident and given
a routine x-ray examination when first admitted to the
clinic. What critical observations do you make on this
radiograph?

→ 192

(a) What methods could you use for sex differentiation in these two birds?

(b) Would you suggest any laboratory tests be carried out on the bird on the left because of its abnormal feathering?

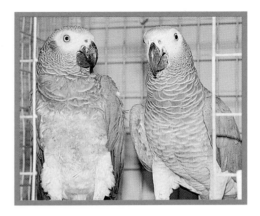

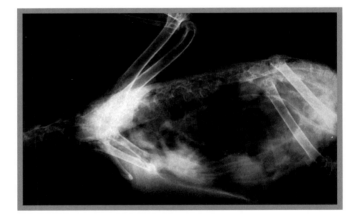

↑ 193

This is a laterolateral radiograph of a blue and gold macaw. The owner reported that the bird was showing weakness, anorexia, weight loss, and diarrhea with undigested food in the feces for the previous 2 weeks. The bird had no contact with any other bird during the previous 6 months.

(a) What is your provisional diagnosis?

(b) What are your differential diagnoses?

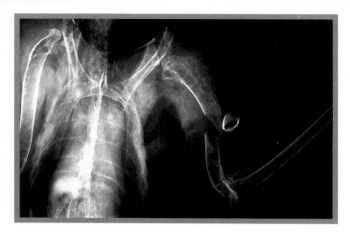

↑   **194**

(a)   What kind of fracture can you see in this ventrodorsal view of a radiograph of a sparrow-hawk *(Accipiter nisus)?*

(b)   What would you consider to be an adequate treatment?

(c)   What factors should be taken into account when keeping this bird during the period of convalescence?

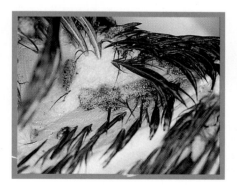

←   **195**

The owner of a flock of pheasants reports that his birds have become highly nervous and are showing dull plumage and reduced growth rates. On examination of several of these birds, you find the changes apparent in the illustration.

(a)   What do you see?

(b)   What do you know about this condition?

(c)   What action should you take?

→ **196**

This illustration was made at postmortem examination of a 30-year-old gray parrot *(Psittacus erithacus)* that died suddenly without antemortem clinical signs.

(a) Do you notice anything that indicates possible abnormality and would lead to a tentative diagnosis as to the cause of death?

(b) How would you confirm your diagnosis?

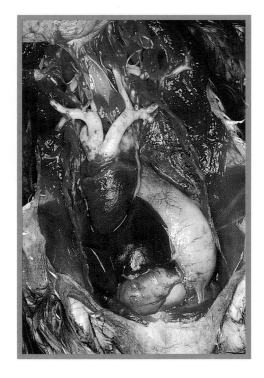

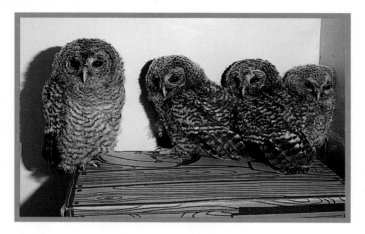

↑   **197**

These four owls were brought into the clinic by three different groups of people, all of whom said they had found these birds by the side of woodland paths when they were out walking. All thought that the birds were either injured, ill, or lost.
(a) What is the species of these birds?
(b) Can you make some assessment of their age?
(c) How has this relatively common situation occurred?
(d) What should these people be advised to do with these owls?

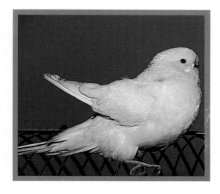

←   **198**

This budgerigar *(Melopsittacus undulatus)* looks abnormally "puffed up." It has a ruptured air sac, probably the clavicular air sac.
(a) How would you diagnose this condition?
(b) What is the exact extent of the clavicular air sac?
(c) How would you deal therapeutically with this condition?

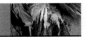

→ 199

This pendulous, bulbous structure was seen attached to the rump (pyga) of a budgerigar *(Melopsittacus undulatus)*.

(a) What are your differential diagnoses?

(b) How would you deal with this lesion therapeutically?

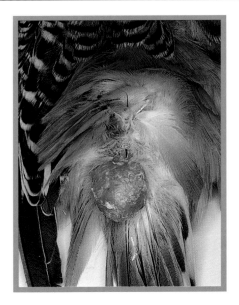

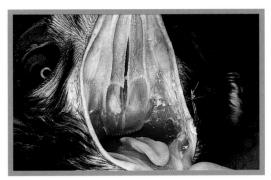

↑ 200

This illustration is of the oral cavity of a buzzard *(Buteo buteo)*.

(a) What significant lesions do you see?

(b) What are your differential diagnoses?

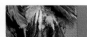

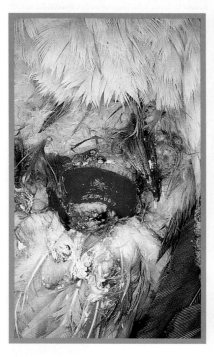

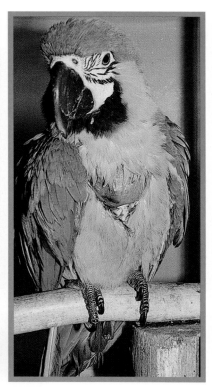

↑ 201

This illustration shows the ventral aspect of the caudal abdomen of an African grey parrot *(Psittacus erithacus)*.

(a) Comment on what you see.

(b) What is the cause of this condition?

↑ 202

This young blue and gold macaw *(Ara ararauna)* was presented with a prominent dark-colored (necrotic appearing) swelling in the region of the thoracic inlet. The bird was still being handfed and had over the previous few days become reluctant to take food.

(a) What is your tentative diagnosis?

(b) How would you treat this condition?

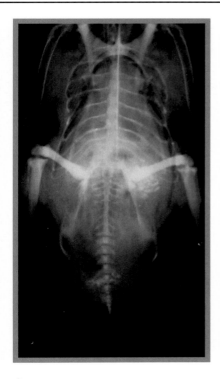

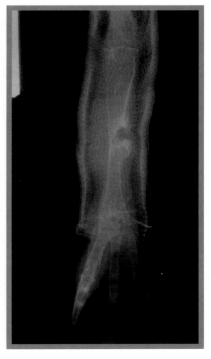

↑ **203**

This is the radiograph of an 18 month old female duck that was presented in a collapsed condition and died 48 hours later. The legs were not fully extended before radiography. What information can be gained from this radiograph?

↑ **204**

This is the dorsoventral projection of the left foot of a northern goshawk *(Accipiter gentilis gentilis)*. The lesion has been temporarily stabilized by encasing in an external splint.

(a) Describe the lesion on the lateral surface of the tarsometatarsus.

(b) What is the possible etiology?

(c) How long this has taken to occur?

(d) What is the most appropriate surgical procedure for dealing with this lesion?

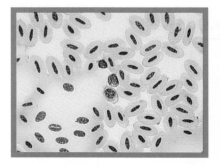

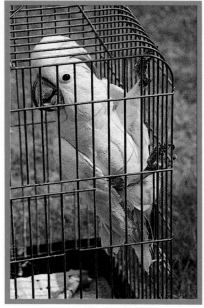

↑ **205**

This is a blood smear from a white stork *(Ciconia ciconia)*. (Giemsa stain; × 1000.) (Courtesy Dr Balks.)

(a) Exactly classify the single cell in the center of this photomicrograph and explain your answer.

(b) What are the most reliable characteristics for identifying lymphocytes? What are the most reliable features in this particular blood smear?

(c) What proportion of the leukocytes do lymphocytes normally compose in avian blood?

(d) What has happened to the erythrocytes in the left lower quadrant of the image?

↑ **206**

How would you proceed in catching this bird for examination?

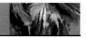

→ **207**

These are the feet of a wild European kestrel *(Falco tinnunculus)* that was found sitting apathetically on the ground.
(a) Describe the lesions.
(b) What might have caused this damage?
(c) What further examination apart from visual inspection would you consider necessary?

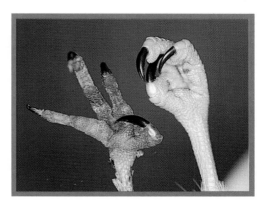

→ **208**

This budgerigar *(Melopsittacus undulatus)* had a history of lameness in its left leg. What is your plan of investigation?

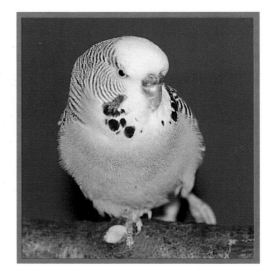

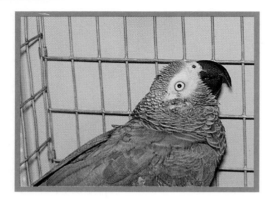

↑ **209**

This African gray parrot *(Psittacus erithacus)* shows ataxia, slight opisthotonus, and episodic convulsions.

(a) What condition often is responsible for these signs in gray parrots?

(b) How would you deal with this problem?

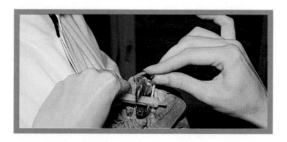

↑ **210**

(a) Comment on the method of restraint and the use of a plastic syringe for examining this parrot's mouth.

(b) What other methods could be used for this examination?

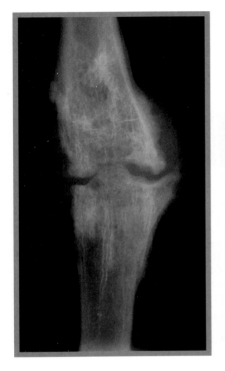

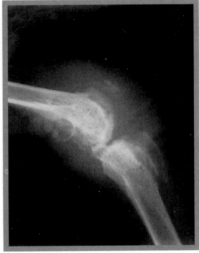

↑ **211, A, B**

These are ventrodorsal **(A)** and laterolateral **(B)** radiographs of a domestic goose *(Anser anser)* that had a noticeably hot, swollen intertarsal joint and was severely lame.

(a) What information can you derive from these radiographs?
(b) What are the most likely predisposing factors?
(c) Can anything be done therapeutically to relieve this condition?
(d) What is the prognosis?

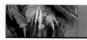

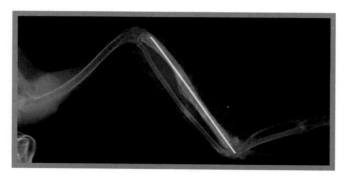

↑ 212

This is the radiograph of the radius and ulna of a tawny owl *(Strix aluco)*. The bird previously had a fracture of these two bones, which was pinned by a veterinarian. Although both fractures have healed, the pin is interfering with the action of the ulna carpal joint. This bird was referred to a consultant veterinarian for removal of the pin in hope that the bird would regain functional use of the joint and be able to fly again. How would you proceed with treatment?

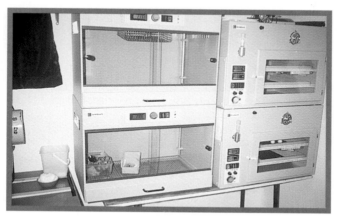

↑ 213

What do you know about the conditions for the artificial hatching of psittacine chicks?

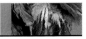

→ **214**
This African gray parrot *(Psittacus erithacus)* chick has an obvious problem with its legs.
(a) What do you observe?
(b) What is the cause of this condition?
(c) Can anything be done to alleviate this condition?

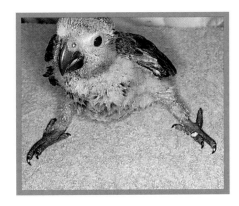

→ **215**
This bird, kept in a zoologic garden, is unwell and spends most of its time in recumbency.
(a) What sort of bird is this?
(b) How many species are there in the genus, and from which geographic location and habitat does it come?
(c) How would you proceed to perform a full clinical examination?

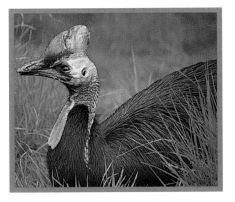

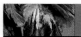

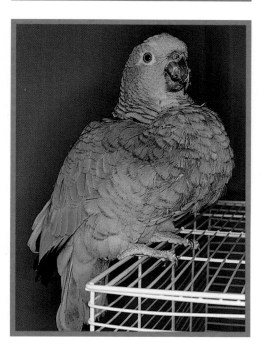

← 216

This culture of *Aspergillus niger* was obtained from a swab taken from the oral cavity of a psittacine bird. What factors should you consider when interpreting this laboratory result?

← 217

This blue-fronted Amazon parrot *(Amazona aestiva)* presented with a prominent, firm-feeling swelling of the neck. When palpated, the temperature of the skin did not feel elevated nor did the skin look erythremic. The bird had no problems feeding or breathing.
(a) How would you investigate this problem?
(b) What is the possible etiology?

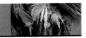

→ 218

This festive Amazon parrot *(Amazona festiva)* has obviously abnormal plumage. It was in good bodily condition, even slightly overweight, and showed no other clinical signs. The owner said the bird received a good mixed diet of seed and fruit. A clinical profile did not indicate liver or kidney disease, and routine screening for infections such as aspergillosis was negative.

(a) Comment on the abnormalities.
(b) What is a possible etiology for this condition?
(c) What therapeutic measures would you suggest?

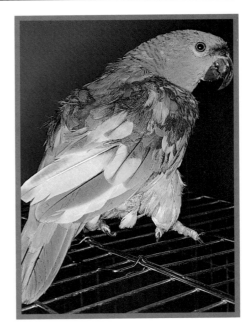

→ 219

(a) What is abnormal about this bird?
(b) What do you know about this condition in birds?
(c) Is there any treatment?

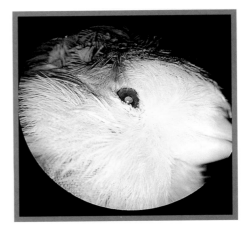

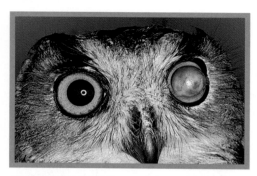

← **220, A, B**

(a) Describe exactly the lesion you see in the keratopathy exhibited by this Eurasian eagle owl *(Bubo bubo)*.

(b) Considering the species of the bird, what is the most likely etiology for this lesion?

(c) What line of therapy would you suggest?

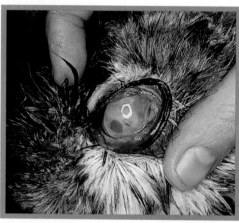

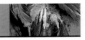

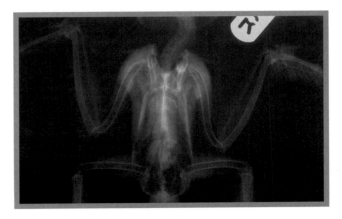

↑   **221**
This is the radiograph of a sparrowhawk *(Accipiter nisus)*
presented as a road traffic casualty.
(a)   What is your diagnosis?
(b)   What line of treatment would you adopt?
(c)   What is the prognosis for this bird?

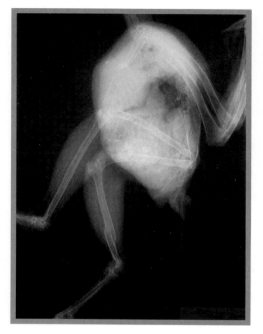

← 222

This is the laterolateral radiograph of a tawny owl *(Strix aluca)* presented as a road traffic casualty. The bird was concussed, but when it recovered it appeared and behaved quite normally.

(a) What lesions do you see in this bird?

(b) Is there a mass of foreign bodies in the abdomen?

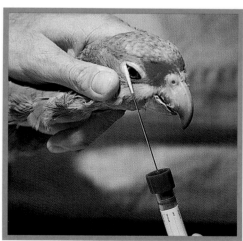

← 223

This newly acquired Amazon parrot *(Amazona* sp.) is having a swab taken from the eye for microbiologic examination. The bird presented with a conjunctivitis, was sneezing, and had a nasal discharge.

(a) What etiologies would you consider?

(b) What other laboratory tests would you carry out?

(c) What are the zoonotic implications of this condition?

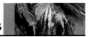

➜ **224**
(a) Identify the parasite shown in this illustration of a blood smear taken from a European kestrel *(Falco tinnunculus)*. (Giemsa; ×1000.)
(b) Does this parasite have any pathologic significance?
(Courtesy Dr. Piera de Palma.)

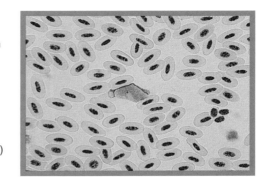

➜ **225**
This red-tailed hawk *(Buteo jamaicensis)* was presented by a falconer with a tumor of the lower eyelid.
(a) How would you handle and investigate this problem in such a powerful raptor?
(b) What type of neoplasms are most likely to involve this region of the bird's anatomy?

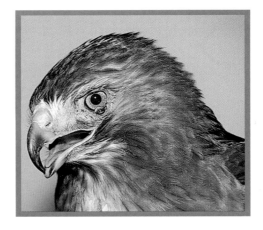

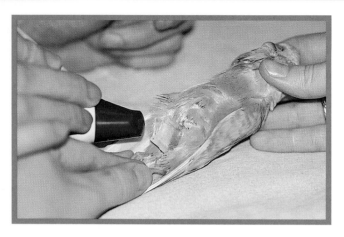

↑ 226
What are the practical indications for the use of
ultrasonography in avian practice?

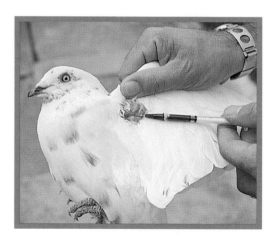

← 227
(a) Which vein is being
used for blood
collection in this bird?
(b) What problems are
you likely to
encounter using this
vein?
(c) Which other veins can
be used?
(d) How much fluid blood
can be withdrawn or
injected
intravenously?

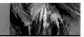

→ 228

This budgerigar nestling *(Melopsittacus undulatus)*, which was only a few days old, died with a massively distended abdomen.

(a) What are your differential diagnoses?

(b) What are your reasons for these?

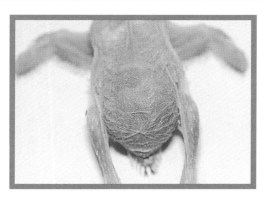

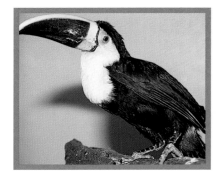

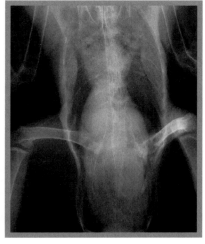

↑ 229, A, B

A, This Cuviers toucan *(Ramphastos cuvieri)* was chronically lame on its right leg. **B,** The laterolateral radiograph of the bird's leg is illustrated.

(a) What do you see on the radiograph?

(b) What is your diagnosis?

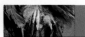

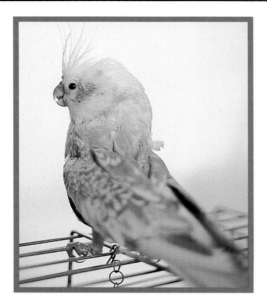

↑   **230**
This cockatiel appears to have a grossly
swollen neck and a swollen dorsal caudal
area of the skull. On palpation the swelling
felt gas filled. The bird was otherwise
normal.
(a)   What is the possible etiology of this
      lesion?
(b)   How would you confirm your
      diagnosis?
(c)   How would you treat this lesion?

Picture Tests Answers

1 (a) A, West African tropical rainforest variety of the crowned crane *(Balearica pavonima)*. **B,** This is Hautleb's tauraco *(Tauraco hautloubi)*.

(b) Feather color is produced by pigmentation, structural colors, or a combination of both. *Structural colors* result from the physical properties of the feather surface, which cause diffraction of the various components of the spectrum that form white light. For example, blue colors result from the reflection of blue light, which has a short wave length, while the other colors are absorbed. The following are the feather pigment colors:

• *Melanins* are produced by melanocytes located in the epidermis as in mammals. These pigments help produce black, gray, brown, or even dull yellow coloring. Melanins are produced in the body, and their production may be affected by a hepatopathy or deficiency of essential amino acids.

• *Carotenoids* are responsible for red, orange, and yellow feather coloration.

• *Carotenes* and *xanthophylls* are absorbed from the diet (e.g., carrots, green foods, paprika, some invertebrates). The degree of dietary absorption is genetically determined.

• Porphyrins are metabolic products and influence red, brown, and true green pigmentation.

• Turacoverdin, a green pigment, is unique to the forest tauracos (e.g., *Tauraco musophagidae*).

• Turacin (containscopper) is another pigment produced by only some tauracos and results in a red color.

(c) Diseases affecting feather growth may also alter the feather structure, thereby influencing their color. Alternatively, metabolic disease or dietary deficiency may affect the color of plumage.

2 (a) These are barn owls *(Tyto alba)*.

(b) In raptorial species the hatching of the eggs is not synchronous as in the case of most Passeriformes and precocial species. Consequently, fledgling barn owls are approximately 2 days apart in hatching, subsequent development, and stage ofinitial molt.

(c) Molting is a natural process in birds during which worn or unsuitable feathers (and also sometimes other keratin structures, such as the scales of the skin, the comb, and wattles) are periodically shed. During molting, most birds can still fly. However, although no naked, unfeathered areas of the body are visible, body insulation is less efficient. Many waterfowl, grebes (Podicipedidae), divers (loons) (Gaviidae), cranes (Gruidae), and rails (Rallidae) molt all their flight feathers at the same time so that they are flightless for up to 28 days. Some female hornbills molt while walled up in their nest and are fed by the male bird. Similarly, the female sparrowhawk molts while incubating her eggs and being fed by the male. Molting places a considerable stress on the bird. Not only are body heat and energy lost through less efficient insulation but the amount of protein required for feather replacement is substantial; it can be 25% of total body protein requirements. During molting the bird needs rest to conserve energy, and it is more vulnerable both to predators and infectious disease.

(d) The frequency of molting varies with the species. Psittacines molt continuously, with a tendency to peak periods in the spring and autumn and taking 8 to 9 months to renew all their plumage. Malnourished birds may take much longer. Many species that normally inhabit temperate climates molt regularly twice yearly in line with their breeding or migra-

129

tory seasons. The large raptors must be able to continue to fly and hunt; therefore they molt continuously but may take 2 years to replace all their feathers.

Control of molting is complex and varies with species. Also, the pattern of molting sometimes is different between males and females of the same species. High blood levels of estrogen and prolactin tend to inhibit molt, while increased thyroxin, progesterone, and testosterone increase molting. In some species, increasing the photoperiod of daylight hours may decrease the molt, while in others the reverse is true. Good nutrition with adequate levels of protein with sulphur-containing amino acids, sufficient energy, and vitamin A are also essential.

3 **(a)** The overall condition of the integument, including the plumage, may give an indication of the bird's health. For example, many infectious diseases, such as chlamydiosis, result in nonspecific disorders such as dull unkempt plumage with lost and broken feathers. The diagnostic aim should always be to establish the primary underlying disease. Therefore, if chlamydiosis is suspected, samples for laboratory examination (i.e., blood and swabs from the conjunctiva, cloaca, and fecal samples) should be obtained. A Coomb's test can indicate a positive and/or rising titer. Pooled fecal samples harvested over a period of several consecutive days can be checked by polymerase chain reaction (PCR) DNA laboratory test for the presence of *Chlamydia* organisms. A full hematologic screen may also help in indicating the underlying disease condition.

(b) The abnormal feathering will improve after treatment of the underlying *primary* disease and also improving the bird's nutritional status, particularly regarding the vitamin and amino acid intake.

4 **(a)** Hyperkeratosis is very common in the mature or aged canary. It is also seen in other Passeriforms, including mynah birds. It has been observed in a single case in a northern goshawk *(Accipiter gentilis gentilis)* and is documented as occurring in ostriches *(Struthio camelus)* as a result of biotin and pantothenic acid deficiency.

(b) In the canary many cases are due to the *Knemidokoptes* mange mite, and others may be related to nutritional or genetic factors. The exact etiology is not always known.

(c) Clinically the increase in diameter of the tarsometatarsus may necessitate the removal of a constricting ring. Also, with increasing severity, the hyperkeratitis may encircle the toe(s) and cause an inflammatory reaction. Lameness and an inability to perch properly are often described by owners.

(d) Treatment consists of daily soaking the hyperkeratotic material in an oily substance and careful removal of the hyperkeratotic scales with forceps. A change of diet may also be indicated.

5 **(a)** In wild birds, necrosis of the foot or leg may be seen after trauma caused by traps, bone fractures, or, as in the case of this particular bird, an electrical injury.

(b) In many cases this results in an inability to survive in the wild. Although raptors may continue to be able to catch prey, buzzards are relatively heavy birds and eventually develop "bumblefoot" on the unaffected but weight-bearing side.

6 **(a)** This bird has almost certainly lost the lower part of its leg by amputation as a result of a constricting ligature of monofilament nylon fishing line. It could of course have lost the foot through some other traumatic incident. Because the traumatized leg was continually being immersed in seawater it would have been kept relatively free of infection and the bird would have been able to spend much of its time roosting on the water.

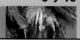

(b) This bird appears to be in good condition. It can probably survive quite well because gulls have a varied diet, feeding on many marine organisms and hawking for insects, carrion, garbage, and, occasionally, even small rodents.

How well a bird survives in the wild with one leg will to some extent depend on its size (see the answer for Fig. 5) but will depend even more on its lifestyle. Waders, even some small species, are severely disabled, but small perching birds such as wrens (Troglodytidae) and thrushes (Turdidae), which hop along the ground in search of food, will fare better than pipits and wagtails (Motacillidae), which run or walk briskly.

7 (a) The clinical signs are typical of articular gout, which is also seen in other species. The distal joints of the legs show typical yellow nodules formed by collections of uric acid crystals, or tophi, which resemble subcutaneous abscesses.

(b) There is some doubt as to the exact etiology of this condition, but it has been suggested that when plasma uric acid levels rise slightly above the level of the solubility of sodium urate (because of renal disease) then uric acid crystals are deposited in the coldest parts of the body (the distal leg joints). The solubility of sodium urate depends on temperature and on plasma sodium concentration.

(c) Treatment consists of reduced dietary protein, increased energy level, and increased vitamin A and vegetable intake. Many cage birds are deficient in vitamin A; this deficiency has a detrimental effect on the viability of all epithelia. Reduce calcium, phosphorus, magnesium, sodium, and vitamin D3 intake, because excessive amounts of all of these can lead to renal mineralization and exacerbate the condition. Increase the intake of the water-soluble B vitamins, because they may be lost with polyuria. Many renal diseases are bacterial in origin, and therefore antibiotic therapy should always be administered.

Allopurinol, which reduces the production of uric acid by the liver, has been used. However, it may result in the deposition of xanthine and hypoxanthine in the renal tubules and therefore should be used with caution.

8 (a) This is Pacheco's disease, caused by a herpesvirus. Conures are often asymptomatic carriers, and New World parrots are more susceptible than Old World parrots. Yellowish feces are one sign of a hepatopathy that could be caused by Pacheco's virus.

(b) Confirmation of diagnosis is by postmortem examination and culture of the virus, which can be identified by enzyme-linked immunosorbent assay (ELISA) and immunofluorescence.

(c) Treatment in high-risk cases is by vaccination (available in the United States). However, vaccination protection takes at least 10 days for effective immunity. Acyclovir (a human drug) given orally has been reported to reduce mortality. The parental administration of this drug is not recommended. Separate diseased birds, enforce rigid quarantine, and thoroughly clean and disinfect the premises. Chlorhexidine or Virkon disinfectant can be used in the drinking water to reduce the risk of viral spread and replication of the virus in the enteric mucosa.

Sick birds should be kept in a warm and quiet environment and fed an adequate diet, ensuring that there are optimum levels of zinc and vitamins A, E, and B. Supplementary ascorbic acid also may help. Many birds that recover can become latent carriers and a source of infection to newly acquired birds.

9, 10 (a) These signs are typical of group 3 paramyxovirus infection, not uncommon amongst *Neophema* and *Platycercus* spp. of parrots. There may also be other associated clinical signs (eye lesions and nasal exudate), although not evident in this particular case. The abnormal

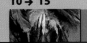

feces are due to the typical concurrent pancreatitis. Birds may also have an increased appetite.

(b) Acyclovir, as used for herpesvirus infections, is not effective with paramyxoviruses. An effective vaccine for turkeys (with reduced egg production) against group 3 paramyxoviruses is available. However, it is suggested that the relevant government disease control authority be contacted before using the vaccine on parrots.

Treatment and control of an outbreak is as described for Pacheco's virus in the answer to Fig. 8.

11 Nebulization therapy is an effective and practical means of treating diseases of the respiratory tract, skin, or feathers that are more difficult to manage on a regular or continuous basis by other methods of therapy. Vapor particles must be between 0.5 to 5.0 μ in diameter so that the medication will penetrate all parts of the respiratory tract. A great advantage of nebulization is that handling of the patient (often untamed birds) and the resulting stress are minimized. Also, staff are protected from inhaling medications and from zoonotic risks. Furthermore, side effects that may result in iatrogenic feather disorders (as may occur with ointments) are avoided.

Because there is no systemic effect with nebulization, this method is contra-indicated in those cases suspected to be suffering from a systemic infection.

Repeat treatment should be once or twice daily for approximately 15 minutes, for several days or, if necessary, weeks.

12 A needle biopsy should be obtained for histopathology to differentiate neoplastic from inflammatory lesions caused by microorganisms. Various neoplasms have been documented as occurring in the integument of birds. The most common are xanthomas, fibrosarcomas, carcinomas, hemangiomas, and hemangiosarcomas. The particular case illustrated was a fibrosarcoma, and the wing was amputated.

13 (a) With magnification it would be possible to see that there is damage to the feather vane caused by feather mites.

(b) A magnifying glass is usually all that is required, although a low-magnification dissecting microscope makes the task easier.

14 (a) This insect is a member of the family Hippoboscidae, commonly known as *flat* or *louse flies*. Some have wings and other species are wingless. When found on sheep they are referred to as *sheep keds*.

(b) Many species of wild birds carry this parasite, particularly the Hirundinidae (i.e., swallows and martins).

(c) This arthropod sucks blood and is thought to transmit Haemoproteus and trypanosomes. Hippoboscids can be a particular problem to young pigeons.

15 (a) This arthropod is a species of *Dermanyssus*, or red mite. These mites are not necessarily red; they can appear black or even buff colored.

(b) These mites spend most daylight hours off the bird and breeding in the crevices of woodwork, in cracks and inaccessible spaces of the cage, or in the mews of captive hawks. They usually migrate onto the perching bird at night. All permanent external parasites tend to leave a dying bird, possibly because they detect a drop in body temperature.

(c) They are found on all species of birds and suck blood. Cases of massive infestation may result in severe anemia and death. Infestation is most serious in young birds and those

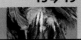

weakened from other causes. Less severely affected birds show intense pruritus and restlessness, leading to loss of condition.
(d) These mites usually are found only on captive hawks.

16 **(a)** This is most likely a bacterial infection subsequent to a bite or foreign body penetration that has resulted in an abscess pushing the horny keratin of the beak and tissues lining the roof of the mouth away from the underlying bone.
In this particular case the infection was caused by *Escherichia coli* and an inability to close the mouth, so that prehension was impossible. Surprisingly, the initial cause was foreign body penetration by a feather barb.
(b) The abscess should be opened surgically and an appropriate antibiotic administered both parentally and locally, for a minimum of 5 to 10 days.
Treatment is complicated because there is a close adhesion of the epidermal tissue to the bone in this region, with little if any subcutaneous tissue. Consequently, the blood supply is disrupted and the prognosis is questionable.

17 **(a)** This is a female specimen of the crossbill *(Loxia curvirostra),* a bird of Western Europe. The species is sexually dimorphic. The female bird is olive green and the male brick-red. The intensity of color increases with age and also with color feeding in captive specimens (i.e., increased dietary carotene as in carrots).
(b) In both sexes the young are born with a normal-appearing beak that crosses over (either to the left or right) when the bird is about 7 weeks old. The young bird is unable to feed itself on the normal diet of pine seeds until the beak is crossed.
(c) The upper eyelid is slightly swollen, and there is a suspicion of dried exudate around the whole eye at the angle of the mouth and over the cheek of the bird. These lesions could be due to Avipoxvirus infection or to *Knemidokoptes* species infection. In crossbills this mite infection is most commonly seen on the legs but does occur on the head.

18 **(a)** This bird is a Waldapp ibis, or Northern bald ibis *(Geronticus eremita),* once common in Central and Eastern Europe but now nearly extinct in the wild. Remnant populations remain in North Africa and the Eastern Mediterranean. The survival of the species is maintained by several European zoos.
(b) The feathering and skin on this bird's head is normal for this species. However, it has broken the tip of its upper beak.
(c) This bird delicately picks up prey (e.g., grasshoppers, beetles, lizards, frogs, fish, and occasionally small mammals or even nestling birds) with its highly sensitive beak; its prehension of moving prey items will be affected by the damaged beak. Although a bird such as this will survive in a zoo situation where it can be fed on minced beef with supplementary vitamins and where the upper and lower beaks can be trimmed to the same length, it would not survive in its natural habitat.

19 **(a)** This abnormality, known as *mandibular prognathism,* is most likely to be caused in adult birds by trauma to the articulations of either upper or lower beak, or both, or to the germinative regions of the keratin. In fledglings and young birds the condition may be congenital, as a result of faulty incubation; may be caused by malnutrition, as in metabolic bone disease; or may be genetic in origin. The consequence of the defect is that the keratin of the distal extremities of both upper and lower beak continues to grow without being worn down by the opposing beak and so maintained in shape. Ultimately, this affects prehension and bodily condition.

(b) The beak can of course be clipped and ground into shape regularly, but this does not provide a permanent solution.

Surgery aims to change the direction of force of the maxillary beak, so that it comes to overlap and impinge on the distal growing tip of the mandibular beak. This objective is achieved by encasing the distal end of the maxillary beak in acrylic prosthetic extension (dental acrylic or technovite), which overlaps the mandibular beak. Both prosthesis and lower beak can be trimmed and ground into shape. However, if too much is removed from the lower beak, the corrective force on the articulation will be lessened. The prosthesis is anchored with cyanomethacrylate (bone cement) after circular grooving of the upper beak to provide a firmer hold. Drilling and the use of fine stainless steel wire or mesh may also be necessary in larger birds to increase adhesion. Some postoperative pain can be controlled by nonsteroidal antiinflammatory drugs (e.g., carprofen). As the underlying keratin grows the prosthesis will gradually loosen and require periodic replacement. Treatment may take 6 months.

20 (a) Clinically there is often pruritus of the entire body surface accompanied by disturbances of feather growth and pigmentation. There may also be inflammatory reactions of the dermis, resulting in an acanthosis. The feather follicles and epidermis may also be inflamed. Feather loss usually starts in one area and gradually spreads, with yellow exudative, crusty vesicles appearing under the wings, and progresses to affect the entire thoracic and abdominal plumage. Because the respiratory tract can soon become involved (through the bird preening), these infections are often fatal as a result of systemic infection.

(b) Dermatomycosis (caused by *Trichophyton, Rhodotorula, Mucor,* and *Cladosporium* organisms) is rare in birds. Budgerigars and canaries with an area of thick, gray, flaky, dusty skin occurring on any part of the body have been documented. The fungi are found in the keratinized layers of the epidermis and produce a variety of inflammatory reactions, but the massive destruction of feather follicles, similar to the necrotic folliculitis of mammalian hair follicles, does not often occur in birds. Mycotic infection in captive birds is usually secondary to poor hygiene and faulty husbandry. *Aspergillus* spp. (e.g., *Aspergillus niger* and *Aspergillus fumigatus*) are probably the most common mycotic, nonspecific pathogens isolated from the plumage of captive birds, although *Mucor* spp. and *Penicillium* spp. are sometimes cultured. Small psittacines and zoologic species often have massive infections of the entire skin and plumage with *Mucor* spp., which can result in severe pruritus.

(c) Diagnosis can be confirmed by microbiologic culture and serology if systemic infection is suspected.

(d) Therapy should consist of the topical application of amphotericin as a cream or the careful use of enilconazol daily for a minimum of 2 weeks. Vitamin A should be given initially by injection and then supplemented orally after the vitamin A content of the diet has been determined.

Management faults such as low humidity and lack of bathing facilities, particularly for tropical birds, should receive attention. In the case of pet birds, spraying with a weak solution (1 part in 380) of chlorhexidine often has a salutary effect. If the respiratory tract is involved, oral treatment with itraconazole or ketoconazole should be instituted.

21 (a) Polyomavirus infection affects many species of psittacines and is one cause of budgerigar fledgling disease.

(b) In the acute phase, when newly hatched budgerigars are affected, mortality is high. In somewhat older fledglings there is symmetric loss of flight feathers and overall poor feather development. About 10% of cases exhibit signs of central nervous system involvement, ascites, and hepatitis. There is massive virus replication within the liver. Histologically, large basophilic intranuclear bodies are found in all affected organs (i.e., most of the viscera and the skin) together with partial or complete degeneration of the feather follicles.

(c) Surviving birds do not thrive, and feather dystrophies continually occur. Older fledglings that lose only their flight feathers are referred to as "runners" and are said to have "French molt."

(d) Controlling infection in an aviary requires thorough cleansing and disinfection, depopulation, and cessation of breeding.

22 (a) These signs are typical of psittacine beak and feather disease. This condition was first recognized in wild cockatoos in Australia during the early 1970s. It is now a global problem affecting many other psittacine species. The cause is an immunosuppressive nonenvelope DNA virus placed in the taxon Circoviridae.

(b) Adolescent to mature birds are affected with progressive symmetric feather loss involving the entire plumage, including the head. Affected birds eventually become flightless. The feathers become brittle and are easily plucked. As the disease proceeds there is increasing feather dystrophy, with persistent feather sheaths (often with blood-filled quills, particularly on the head) and misshapen, thickened, and curled feathers, many showing encircling constrictions of the quill. In more advanced cases, beak and nail deformities become apparent. The beak can become elongated or malformed, and the distal extremity can become necrotic. This chronic condition can persist for months or even a few years. Death caused by secondary infection as a result of immunosuppression and impairment of core body thermoregulation is the result. However, in some species (e.g., budgerigars *[Melopsittacus undulatus]*) the head is not always affected, and infected birds do not always die. In vasa parrots *(Coracopsis* spp.) the black plumage becomes progressively white.

23 (a) This particular bird was presumed to be suffering from hypovitaminosis E and associated muscular dystrophy, which has been described as being particularly common in lutino cockatiels. The loss of movement in the wings and the marked clamping of them to the underlying sternum is thought to be due to muscle fibrosis.

(b) In this case there was very little response to injections of vitamin E and selenium, and no protozoal parasites could be demonstrated in the fresh droppings. The owner elected for euthanasia and would not consent to a postmortem examination; therefore histopathology could not confirm the diagnosis.

(c) It is said that an infection with *Giardia* or *Hexamita* may produce a malabsorption of vitamin E. Deficiency may also occur in improperly stored, rancid food.

24 (a) This condition is variously known as "angel wing," "straw wing" or "flip wing." It results from a valgus deformity of the growing carpometacarpal bones, which become rotated laterally to approximately 180 degrees, causing the primary flight feathers to stick out when the wing is folded at rest to the body. These birds are flightless. The condition occurs in fledglings in both wild and captive waterfowl and is most common in the larger species (i.e., geese and swans). It also occurs in some psittacine species (budgerigars, macaws, and conures).

Various etiologies have been suggested for this condition, but it is likely that no one single cause produces the abnormality and the condition is multifactorial. Contributing factors may be of genetic origin or related to incubation and hatching problems or malnutrition. Diets with too high a level of protein (in excess of 18%), calcium and phosphorus imbalance, and hypovitaminosis D_3 may result in too rapid a growth of blood-filled (and relatively heavy) flight feathers being carried on inadequately mineralized bone. As in some other cases of metabolic bone disease, not all members of a clutch may develop the condition.

(b) Diagnosis is by physical examination, when the flexion and extension of all the wing joints may be found to be normal or abnormal. There also may be an abnormal laxity in the joints and some subluxation of the tendon of the propatagium over the carpal region. Radiography is only of value in advanced cases.

(c) Treatment consists of splinting and the use of a figure 8 bandage changed every 3 days. This may be effective on younger fledglings showing very early signs of abnormality. In more mature birds with pronounced bone deformity, osteotomy of the major metacarpal bone is performed. The distal segment is then rotated around an intramedullary pin, which is left in place for 6 to 8 weeks, until the bone heals. The wing is bandaged in the normal position, and the bandage is changed regularly. The chances of the bird being able to fly again are about 50%.

25 (a) The premaxillary beak is obviously overgrown at its distal extremity and should be trimmed to its normal length, a process known to the falconer as *coping*. This is carried out using sharp (veterinary) nail clippers or garden shears for larger birds. Coping is finished with sandpaper, an emery board (as used for fingernails), or a fine file. When reshaping the beaks of falcons, care should be taken to preserve the tomial teeth on the cutting edge of the upper beak and the corresponding notches on the mandibular beak. These are used to kill as the bird bites the neck of prey. These teeth may also be used to bite up the bones of prey.

(b) Overgrowth of the horn of the beak in captive raptors often occurs because this is a continuously growing structure requiring constant wear to maintain its true length. This peregrine had been fed on a diet of surplus dead hatchery chicks for a prolonged period, which resulted in very little wear on a beak normally used for tearing more robust flesh and tendon.

(c) A continuous diet of freshly hatched chicks is too high in fat because of unabsorbed yolk in the yolk sac. Some falconers provide their birds with "tiring," a piece of tough meat on which the bird can pull. This not only helps to keep the beak in trim but also strengthens the muscles of the neck and back.

26 The following are differential diagnoses:
• Possible lead poisoning from fishermen's lead sinker weights. Fishing line becomes entangled with underwater vegetation if it cannot be retrieved and it is discarded along with the attached weight. This can be ingested by swans feeding on subaqueous vegetation. Particles of river bottom gravel may be swallowed (to aid the bird's digestion) amongst which may be lead shot left after wildfowling. Both sources of lead are common. No clinical signs are pathonomic, but birds are usually weak, have lost weight, and cannot hold their heads up (the typical S-bend in the swan's neck is lost.) Passage of greenish liquid droppings is common.

In Canada geese *(Branta canadensis)* and the snow goose *(Anser caerulescens)*, cephalic edema is also documented. Diagnosis is by dorsoventral radiography of proventriculus and gizzard, blood chemistry, and hematology. However, lead levels vary and only those above 5 μmol/l are significant. Lead poisoning is not usually acute in onset and is not epidemic.

• Botulism, or so called limberneck, also known in the United States as *western duck disease.* This is commonly caused by type C toxin produced by the obligate anaerobic saprophyte *Clostridium botulinum.* The disease is prevalent in hot (30° to 37° C [86° to 99° F]), dry weather

when water levels are low, water quality deteriorates, and vegetation, invertebrates, and fish die, leaving decaying animal protein and rotting vegetation. Once the bacterium begins to thrive and produce toxin, this toxin is concentrated in blowfly maggots, which are eaten by wildfowl, which in turn die and produce more clostridium and toxin, and so on. Swans are not affected as often as other waterfowl or gulls. The disease tends to be epizootic. Once produced, toxin can remain in uneaten maggots or pupae, which may remain in sediment in water or in soil until colder winter weather ensues. Diagnosis is by the mouse protection test. Serum samples from affected birds are injected into mice, half of which are protected by type-specific antitoxin and half not protected.
• Algal poisoning by *Cyanobacteria* (i.e., blue green algae), which may be associated with botulism. This disease occurs in hot, sunny weather, but not necessarily dry weather. The organisms thrive in eutrophic warm water fed by nutrients from agricultural runoff or urban sewage. The water becomes colored and turbid, causing an algal bloom that may be concentrated by wind at one side or end of static water. Diagnosis largely depends on analysis of the field situation. Unlike botulism (i.e., type C toxin), algal poisoning affects both mammals and birds. In birds the neurotoxin causes eye blinking, excessive salivation, repeated swallowing, central nervous system signs, and rapid death. Algal poisoning tends to be epizootic.
• Many infectious diseases, such as pasteurellosis; possibly Newcastle disease PMV 1 (rare in waterfowl); and salmonella, mycobacteria, and aspergillosis infections, can produce central nervous system signs, but they are not usually so dramatic as those described above.

27 **(a)** Contributing factors include the following:
• Dirty, unhygienic perches possibly covered in abrasive sandpaper
• Perches that are all the same diameter, so that the bird rarely exercises its feet to encourage an active blood supply
• Obesity resulting from overfeeding (food should be rationed)
• Hypothyroidism caused by a lack of iodine, contributing to obesity and retarding healing
• Deficiency of vitamin E (affects muscle activity) or vitamin A (affects the viability of epithelial tissues)
• Deficiency of calcium, although some birds may have access to soluble grit and cuttlefish bone
(b) Treatment is described in the answer to Fig. 56, with the addition of cushioned rubber or polyurethane foam padding on the floor of the cage.

28 A needle biopsy performed, which revealed the swelling to be a lipoma. The lipoma was then carefully dissected out. Healing then occurred by first intention.

29 **(a)** A permanent groove can be seen leading down the beak from the external nares, resulting from a chronic rhinitis, which causes a constant exudation. This persistent rhinorrhea has also partially débrided the surrounding area of feathers. A microbiologic etiologic agent causing respiratory disease is possibly involved.
(b) Recently acquired birds demonstrating signs of respiratory disease should be checked for *Chlamydia psittaci*, mycotic and bacterial organisms, and mycoplasma. Nasal, conjunctival, cloanal, and cloacal (for *Chlamydia*) swabs should be obtained.

30 **(a)** Beak and nail lesions and associated feather dystrophies sometimes occur, especially in canaries, as a result of in-breeding.
(b) This particular bird also showed feather cysts and nail deformities.

31 (a) This is a zebra finch *(Taeniopygia guttata)*.
(b) The crusty, powdery lesion is typical of knemidocoptic mange.
(c) Diagnosis is confirmed by microscopic examination of scrapings cleared in potassium hydroxide.
(d) Regarding treatment, in very small birds a single drop of 1% ivermectin dropped onto the skin at the back of the neck will be absorbed percutaneously, spread throughout the bird's body, and eventually taken up by the mites, which are thus killed. Alternatively, application of a very small amount of petroleum jelly to the lesion is often effective in blocking the respiratory openings of the mites.

32 (a) Apart from the obviously broken distal ends of the feathers, the vanes are not spread normally but are gummed together. This bird has been kept in an undersized cage where it was unable to perch above floor level. Similarly damaged feathers may result when a bird is severely ill and spends most of its time on the ground. In some cases, crowding the number of birds in an unsuitable cage can have the same result. This condition also may be seen in flightless wild birds, that have been "*en route* on foot" for some time.
(b) Prevention in hospitalized birds, particularly those with long tails (e.g., diurnal raptors) is carried out by fitting a tail guard made of old x-ray film or strong brown manila paper kept in place with staples or adhesive tape.

33 The probable cause of this feather dystrophy is a dietary deficiency. Such deficiencies are most often seen in birds requiring a complex and versatile diet. A tentative diagnosis can only be given in such cases after all other possibilities have been excluded. Dietary deficiency should always be considered among the differential diagnoses in birds with such clinical signs as persistent feather sheaths, scaliness of the unfeathered skin, pruritus, feather defects (e.g., stress, hunger, or prey marks), parakeratosis, or hyperkeratosis. Malnutrition is known to result in hyperkeratosis of the skin accompanied by feather loss (e.g., resulting from hypovitaminosis A) and loss of pigmentation with associated parakeratosis (pantothenic acid deficiency). Inadequate iodine in the diet can result in hypothyroidism affecting overall health, including that of the skin. A heavy endoparasitic infection may retard the absorption of nutrients.
In this particular bird the persistence of the feather sheaths responded to vitamin B therapy and the elimination of the endoparasites.

34 Many diseases of farmed ostriches are management related. In this situation the maintenance of an adequate hygienic routine is of prime importance. If this is not carried out, alimentary disorders will regularly occur.
The sawdust bedding on the left side of the illustration may be eaten, resulting in impaction or coprophagia, exacerbating any gastrointestinal infectious problem. Although there is an extractor fan, its breakdown or malfunction could result in the rapid spread of airborne pathogens, particularly aspergillosis if the bedding material was previously damp or dusty, thereby encouraging the production of spores. If wild migratory birds get into this restricted air space, infectious viral diseases are also a possibility. Lastly, injury may occur on the corners of feeding troughs, unprotected glass windows, loose paneling, and so on.

35 (a) The proximal part of the upper beak, the cere, is less densely keratinized but is thick and well vascularized.
(b) Beneath this area lies the craniofacial hinge, where the premaxilla (over which lies the horn of the upper beak) and the nasal bone articulate via a flexible junction with the frontal

bone. This enables the gape of the bird to be increased so that it is able to swallow large portions of the prey.

(c) Scar tissue formation in this region as a result of trauma may reduce the flexibility and range of movement of this articulation and so affect prehension and deglutination of food.

36, 37 (a) In Fig. 36 the bird on the left is holding its head in an abnormally extended position. Both birds, particularly that on the right, are overweight.

(b) These signs indicate thyroid dysplasia and hypothyroidism with associated obesity.

(c) The bird on the left holds its head in such a position because the thyroid gland is enlarged. The outlet of the crop is partially obstructed so that the crop is distended. This is clearly seen in the postmortem illustration. This particular bird might also exhibit a change in voice, which often sounds like a squeaky wheel, as a result of pressure of the enlarged thyroid on the syrinx. Sometimes these cases regurgitate continually, in which case they tend to lose weight rather than become obese.

(d) These birds need supplementary iodine in their drinking water (Lugol's iodine, one drop/20 ml drinking water). Seed should be rationed to reduce energy intake. They should be fed weighed quantities of food twice daily, rather than allowed to feed at will. They should be introduced to a formulated diet, and their level of exercise should be increased.

38 (a) Loss of a claw can occur following a momentous traumatic insult leaving only bone and some germinal epithelium. Aside from trauma, malnutrition, in-breeding, chronic infection resulting from being housed in unhygienic conditions, and frost bite can all result in the loss of a claw in all species.

(b) The whole area must be thoroughly cleansed, preferably with povidone-iodine solution and then covered with a hydrophilic dressing. The dressing should be changed every 6 to 7 days. If the germinal area and bone are allowed to dry, they will become invaded with secondary infection. Parental antibiotics are also recommended.

39 (a) This condition is seen especially in older birds. It begins with baldness on the crown of the head and can progress to symmetric feather loss and nakedness on the neck and shoulder areas. In advanced cases there can be complete alopecia. This can be result of a functional disorder of the gonads. Wild birds housed in unsuitable husbandry conditions can develop a similar type of feather loss, which is also caused by a hormonal disturbance.

(b) Treatment consists of progesterone or testosterone administered parentally once a week for up to 6 weeks. However, diagnostic laboratory tests must first be carried out to make sure the patient does not have any signs of a hepatopathy.

40 (a) Contamination with industrial mineral oil is most commonly seen in marine birds after a massive oil spillage, usually after an accident involving an oil tanker. However, other types of birds can also become affected by various kinds of oil products. For example, the leakage of diesel fuel oil from a farm storage tank into a local water course may affect fresh water birds.

The principal results of mineral oil contamination of birds, the severity of which depends to some extent on the type of oil product, are the following:

• The most obvious effect is external damage to the plumage, eyes, legs and feet, nares, and beak.
• The toxic effect on the mucous membranes of the gastrointestinal tract is a result of contaminant swallowed as the bird attempts to preen itself.
• Damage to the plumage results in hypothermia.
• The bird becomes severely stressed.

(b) Oil-soaked plumage can be cleaned under a continuous stream of warm water (35° to 42° C [95° to 108°]F) with a little added detergent (dishwashing soap). The bird is then dried in a gentle flow of warm air. Machines are now being developed for this purpose and are proving to be less stressful than hand washing.

Attention must be given to counteracting any potential harm to the gastrointestinal tract by the administration of kaolin and charcoal preparations. Possible dehydration must be countered.

Even after the removal of all oil from the plumage the barbules of the feathers may not mesh together properly because of permanent damage, and an effective heat insulation layer is not formed. Some birds may therefore have to be retained until after their next molt.

These birds need an easily digestible diet providing a higher caloric intake and supplemental vitamins and minerals because of possible impaired intestinal absorption.

41, 42 (a) Diagnosis would initially be based on biopsy and histopathologic or cytologic examination, which would reveal the intracytoplasmic inclusions known as *Bollinger bodies* typical of avipox virus infection. This could then be confirmed with viral culture from fecal samples. Serology in pox infections is not very useful.

(b) The cutaneous form of avian pox has been described in over 70 species of birds. At least 17 strains of virus have been identified. Many strains of avipox virus are adapted to single families of birds, and some, such as the pigeon pox virus, are species (or at least genera) specific. Pox lesions may also present as papules or larger epidermal proliferative masses often complicated by secondary infections of bacteria, fungi, or trichomonads. The skin around the head (particularly the commissures of the mouth), beak, and eyelids are the areas generally affected. Although previously this disease was described as affecting only the unfeathered parts of the body, it is now observed on the feathered parts of the skin as well. In these areas an unusual tumorlike form of the disease known as *epithelioma contagiosa* may be exhibited by single birds while others in the flock show the more typical signs. Lesions of the oropharynx may block the esophagus and larynx.

(c) There is no specific antiviral treatment. Vaccination of all in-contact pigeons as soon as a diagnosis has been confirmed will usually control an outbreak within 7 to 10 days. Vaccination should be accompanied by treatment of the secondary infections according to laboratory culture and antibiotic sensitivity testing. Vitamins, particularly vitamin A, should be added to the diet. The premises should be thoroughly disinfected. Because arthropod parasites are believed to act as mechanical vectors, all external parasites on the birds should be eliminated. Mosquitoes may carry and spread the virus by inoculation; therefore any areas of standing water near pigeon lofts should receive attention.

In canaries *(Serinus canarius)* a systemic infection leading to pneumonia but without any cutaneous or oral lesions usually results in sudden death. A vaccine is also available (in the United States) for canaries as a prophylactic measure.

43 (a) This is an Atlantic or Northern gannet *(Sula bassana bassana)*.

(b) The nostrils are entirely closed by cornified cells so that the bird breathes through a gap at the corner of the mouth. The opening can be seen at the ventral end of the S-shaped crack in the upper beak, just rostral to the eye. This gap can be closed when the bird plunge dives to catch fish.

(c) These birds are aggressive, readily striking with beaks that have very sharp, serrated cutting edges that enable the bird to securely hold fish.

(d) Gannets build their nests of seaweed, amongst which may be discarded nylon fishing net or line. The bird takes this as part of the nesting material and becomes entangled in it.

Answers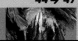

44 (a) In many mynahs these signs occur in advanced cases of hemochromatosis or iron storage disease.
(b) The disease has been documented in many species of birds and also occurs as a genetic defect in humans. In birds it seems that the genetic aspect does not play an important role. Aside from the hill mynah, this is also an important disease in Rothschild's mynah *(Leucopsar rothschildi)*, birds of paradise, quetzals, and the toco toucan *(Ramphastos toco)*, as well as other Ramphastidae (toucans, toucanets, and Aracaris).
Liver histopathology reveals iron deposits in the hepatocytes and Kupffer's cells. A secondary cardiomyopathy may also occur as a result of iron deposits in cardiac cells. The following measures will help to stabilize such a desperately ill bird.
• Hospitalize the bird in a cage where oxygen therapy can be given.
• Consider use of cardiac stimulants in the drinking water, such as digoxin pediatric drops (e.g., Lanoxin PG elixir, 50 μg/ml). The dose in drinking water is 0.013 ml/100 ml drinking water.
• Avoid stressing the bird and keep it quiet and in subdued light.
• Add glucose to the drinking water.
• Consider very careful paracentesis of ascitic fluid to relieve dyspnea.
(c) Long term-therapy consists of regular phlebotomy (1% of body weight/weekly), constantly monitoring the hematologic parameters, and feeding a diet low in iron content (e.g., fruit such as apple, banana, grape, pear, pineapple, or plums, boiled potato, cooked rice, yoghurt, and cooked egg white).

45 (a) These lesions are caused by *Knemidokoptes pilae* mites, which burrow into and feed on the keratin of the skin, causing hyperkeratinization and disfigurement of affected areas. These mites are particularly common in budgerigars, although they will infect other species.
Although the live history is completed entirely within the skin of infected birds, the dust of bird rooms and the nesting areas is often heavily contaminated with mites.
(b) The minute tunnel opening formed by the burrowing mite can easily be seen in the illustration. Lesions may be found anywhere on the body. Pruritus is not a notable feature in the budgerigar, although it may be more evident in other psittacine birds.
(c) Treatment is as described in the answer to Fig. 31. Disfiguring crusts can be carefully softened with liquid paraffin and then gently removed.

46 (a) On physical examination this lesion looks suspiciously like a neoplasm. This was confirmed by radiography and histopathology. It was found to be an osteosarcoma involving the frontal and nasal bones.
(b) Although there was no evidence of metastasis (which is unusual), the lesion was progressive, necessitating eventual euthanasia. Because of the scissor beak, prehension of food was affected.
(c) Surgery of the beak apart from palliative trimming was not justified.

47, 48 (a) These illustrations show emerging feathers that are misshapen, with distorted quills exhibiting constrictions. There is prominent after feather growth without corresponding development of the feather vane. These signs are characteristic of psittacine beak and feather disease.
(b) Diagnosis can be confirmed by histopathology of a skin biopsy fixed in 10% formol saline or by using a DNA probe on a heparinized blood sample. Nevertheless, some birds that are negative for the DNA test are positive on histologic examination and vice versa, particularly those birds showing atypical signs. Consequently, both laboratory tests should be performed to make a firm diagnosis.

Pathohistologically, degenerative signs are seen in the developing contour feather follicles. Often there is epidermal hyperkeratosis and a nonpurulent inflammatory reaction of the feather pulp. Basophilic intracytoplasmic and intranuclear inclusion bodies can be demonstrated in the mononuclear cells of the feather pulp and epidermis.

49 **(a)** This is most likely a case of hypovitaminosis A, which results in a squamous metaplasia of the glands of the mucous membrane, leading to hyperkeratosis. The effect is an apparent abscess filled with sterile, yellowish-white caseous exudate. Other epithelial surfaces in the respiratory, gastrointestinal, and urogenital tracts also are quite likely to be affected.
(b) Differential diagnosis should include avipox lesions, microbiologic abscesses (the above lesion could also be secondarily affected), and possibly candidiasis or trichomoniasis if granulomatous lesions are seen in the oropharynx and are positive on laboratory examination.
(c) Treatment should consist of careful surgical removal of the keratin mass, taking note that the submandibular region is well supplied with blood vessels. Vitamin A should be administered initially parentally, followed by dietary supplementation, 5000 IU/kg q24h for 2 to 4 weeks is the maximum dose (high doses can be toxic). The diet of the bird should be changed in the long term so that it is well balanced and versatile.

50 **(a)** This bird probably has a renal infection, as indicated by the lack of urates in the droppings. Also, its being "off color" for a few days and the loss of weight indicate a possible systemic infection. The legs are innervated by the femoral, obturator, and ischiatic nerves from the lumbosacral plexus and are all closely associated with the kidneys. Any nephritis and swelling of the kidney not only causes pressure on the nerves but may produce an associated neuritis and resultant paresis or paralysis of the legs.
(b) The differential diagnosis is a luxation or subluxation of the vertebral column, particularly between the last thoracic vertebrae and the synsacrum.
(c) Diagnosis of both conditions may be helped by radiography. Intravenous pyelography may indicate a more dense and swollen kidney. To demonstrate luxation, the vertebral column should be "stretched" to reveal any increase in the intravertebral joint space.
Nephrotic cases may show uricemia but more often demonstrate leukocytosis. Occasionally some cases of posterior paresis or paralysis have been found on postmortem examination to be caused by an *Aspergillus* granuloma.

51 **(a)** Aquatic birds kept on an unsuitable substrate (e.g., concrete or tarmacadam) often develop "bumblefoot" lesions, particularly if they are prevented free access to clean water.
(b) In animal rescue centers, rescued birds tend to be overcrowded and both standing and bathing water easily become unhygienic. Astroturf, butyl rubber, or a good expanse of clean grass are preferable roosting surfaces. All surfaces need at least daily hosing, and birds should be allowed to bath frequently in clean water. A large earthenware washing basin or butyl rubber-lined pool in which the water is changed daily and to which chlorhexidine is added is suitable. The birds' diet should contain adequate vitamin A.

52 **(a)** This could of course be a congenital condition. It is most likely caused by the bird having become entangled with fine nylon monofilament fishing line that has acted as a ligature, resulting in amputation.
(b) In the long term this bird would survive in a sanctuary where there is support feeding, but its survival in a wild habitat is doubtful. Because these birds feed mainly on subaqueous vegetation with a little animal matter, such as frogs, worms, small fish, and invertebrates, prehension of sufficient food to maintain health would be difficult.

53 **(a)** This is a cyst with the same etiology as the lesion illustrated in Fig. 49. Such lesions may also be secondarily infected (in this particular case the lesion was sterile).
(b) Differential diagnosis should include a neoplasm and is otherwise as for Fig. 49.
(c) The bird's ability to feed will be severely affected, because most parrots use the tongue for manipulating seeds, nuts, and so on into the correct position for cracking by the beak. Parrots are the only birds that have intrinsic tongue muscles. Once the lesion has been surgically treated, the long-term prognosis is good.

54 A good anamnesis is essential. Was this condition of acute onset or did it develop gradually? Is this a captive or wild bird? If captive, did the keeper notice any other symptoms even over the preceding days or weeks? A careful and systematic physical examination may reveal other signs, such as external trauma to the skin. There may be some neurologic deficit (is the bird's right wing held normally?), paresis, or ataxia. Examine the external ear for signs of inflammatory reaction, and investigate the possibilities of systemic infectious disease. Carefully watch the head for any sign of rhythmic movement in either a horizontal or vertical direction, particularly if the bird is stressed. This may be indicative of nystagmus. Ophthalmic examination may reveal finer regular movements of the fundus. Radiography may show fractures or a unilateral alteration in bone density of the skull. If available, an electro-encephalogram or even magnetic resonance imaging may help to provide a definite diagnosis.

55 **(a)** This cere is normal. In aged male pigeons the dermis often tends to become hyperplastic with a nodular appearance.
(b) Sexual dimorphism is not a reliable guide to gender in pigeons. This cere is a healthy snowy white. If the cere turns even slightly off-white or gray, the clinician should be suspicious of an upper respiratory problem even if there is no overt nasal discharge or other signs.

56 **(a)** This is a case of "bumblefoot," or pododermatitis, a condition linked to stress, obesity, malnutrition, and, particularly in captive raptors, faulty management.
(b) A variety of bacterial organisms can be isolated from these lesions, but *Staphylococcus* spp. are considered a common isolate. Mixed bacterial cultures also can be obtained. The lesion is often associated with excessive trauma to the foot, with puncture or abrasion of the scales of the epidermis allowing the entry of microorganisms. The skin of the foot is in many places adherent to underlying bone so that any swelling resulting from the inflammatory response is restricted. Infection tends to travel along tendon sheaths and other planes of least resistance. The condition can become severe, with deep infection spreading to the joints and leading to eventual septic necrosis of the bone.
(c) Treatment should be directed to improving the diet with the addition of vitamins and minerals, particularly parental vitamin A initially (maximum 20,000 IU/kg IM). If the bird is even slightly overweight, reduce this amount of vitamin A. Increase the bird's exercise to improve the vascular supply to the foot. Cover all perches with an artificial turf product. Keep the bird off all abrasive or gritty surfaces.
The main steps in the basic surgical routine are as follows:
• Incise circularly to remove scab and pus.
• Take swabs for culture and sensitivity.
• Cleanse daily with providone-iodine solution or chlorhexidine and débride.
• Once the wound shows healthy granulation, suture the wound to close or at least reduce in size.
• Dress the wound daily with dermisol cream on nonadherent dressing and bandage the whole foot.

• After granulation, apply Granuloflex hydrophilic dressing and change every 3 days.
• During the whole healing process, support the foot on a well-padded but rigid foot caste (epoxy car repair kit, dental acrylic, Technovite) so that the healing tissues are relieved of pressure.

57 (a) The tip of the phallus is beginning to show signs of drying and early necrosis.
(b) Prolapse of this organ occurs in ducks that are breeding on dry land or that are bullied by dominant ducks. It possibly may be genetic in origin. It is not the result of sexual overindulgence.
Several cases occurring simultaneously may indicate duck viral enteritis (a herpesvirus).
(c) If the prolapse is allowed to continue, necrosis, frostbite, and secondary infection result. Nothing can be done to return the organ to its normal position, and it should therefore be amputated.

58 Papillomaviruses have been found in basophilic intranuclear inclusion bodies in papillomas on the legs and feet exclusively in canaries *(Serinus canaria)* and other finches. These lesions must be differentiated from those caused by knemidocoptic mange mites.
Treatment in the case presented consisted of surgical removal of the papillomas so far as was possible. The prognosis was guarded.

59 (a) The disease is characterized by an irregular and continuous growth of the feather and with a twisting, curling, and splitting of the feather along its long axis. The disease is first noticed soon after fledging, when the chicks begin to develop feathers. Other defects, such as microphthalmia, are also often seen.
(b) The fledglings cannot fly, body heat conservation is impaired, and life expectancy is short. Most birds die at 6 to 8 weeks of age, although survival for as long as 2 years has been documented. The condition is thought to be due to a recessive gene often associated with buff coloring. Known carriers of the gene can be mated so as to produce "feather dusters."

60 (a) Most of the premaxillary bone will have been lost, although the craniofacial hinge is unlikely to have been damaged. Radiography will confirm this.
(b) In this particular bird there will be little regeneration of the horn covering the beak because with no underlying bony proforma on which the beak can reform this part of the beak will not regenerate.
However, parrots that have lost their upper beak often survive quite well by quickly learning to feed on soft food. This is scooped up, using the lower beak like a shovel. Female birds are sometimes fed by male birds. For climbing, parrots without an upper beak learn to compensate by gripping objects (e.g., the bars of the cage) between the mandibular, or lower, beak and the tongue.
The parrot in the illustration survived at least 9 years after the avulsion of its upper beak.

61 (a) This is a subspecies of the gray parrot, *Psittacus erithacus* (timneh). It is slightly smaller and has generally darker plumage than the nominate race.
(b) It inhabits lowland tropical rainforest of West Africa.
(c) Although it is sometimes necessary to apply ointments for the treatment of skin disorders in birds, ointments may cause additional feather loss. Application of ointments may result in pruritus, because feathers in contact with ointment tend to adhere to each other. Because of the bird's constant preening, greasy ointments may get smeared over the whole of the body plumage. In a severe case this can result in marked hypothermia and death, as

in the case of oiled seabirds. For these reasons, the area treated with ointment should be as small as possible. The minimum quantity of ointment should be dabbed on the affected area, preferably with a cotton-tipped applicator. If possible, it is better to use a water-miscible cream or gel preparation. Alternatively, the affected area can be sprayed with the medicine in aqueous solution. Corticosteroids should not be applied to large areas over prolonged a period, because they can, as in the case illustrated, result in skin necrosis and cause undesirable systemic reactions because of percutaneous absorption.

62 This appears to be a dermatitis characterized by epidermal erosion, dermal hyperemia, and transudation or exudation. When this type of lesion is found in the crop or ventral neck area, it is usually due to a factor of faulty management, such as unsuitable types of food cups, that causes constant irritation. The metal or sharp plastic cup edges may cause abrasion and secondary infection of the skin. In this case *Staphylococcus* sp. was the secondary bacterial organism isolated.

63, 64 (a) These pigeons (Fig. 63 is a racing pigeon, and Fig. 64 is a feral pigeon) both show the clinical signs typical of *Paramyxovirus* infection. This is most likely PMV serotype group 1-pigeon, a mutant strain of the original PMV 1 (Newcastle disease virus). Pigeons generally are more resistant to the original virus.
(b) PMV 1-pigeon can also infect chickens, wild raptors, parrots, pheasants (including peafowl), and tauracos. It is carried by house sparrows *(Passer domesticus)* and blackbirds *(Turdus merula)*, which usually do not exhibit clinical signs.
(c) The clinical picture of the bird illustrated in Fig. 63 could be confused with a fractured wing or with a *Salmonella*-induced arthritis. Both of these conditions could be confirmed by radiography or laboratory examination. It should be noted that salmonellosis could also be responsible for central nervous system signs, such as torticollis.

65 (a) This is an unusual case of a budgerigar affected on only the feet and legs with *Knemidokoptes* sp. infestation (see Fig. 45).
(b) Diagnosis can be confirmed by microscopic examination of skin scrapings cleared with potassium hydroxide. The differential diagnoses are nutritional deficiencies, hyperkeratosis, and parakeratosis.

66 (a) Possible differential diagnoses include the following:
• Possibly toxoplasmosis. This is not common in parrots but can cause these clinical signs if the food was contaminated with cat feces. Diagnosis is by histopathology and possibly serology.
• Coccidiosis may cause diarrhea but is unlikely to produce central nervous system signs. Confirmation of diagnosis is by fecal examination.
• Paramyxoviruses cause CNS signs and usually cause yellow-white chalky or waxy feces (see Fig. 10). PMV-3 is also pathogenic for many species of finches. Diagnosis is by histopathology and various laboratory tests.
• Psittacine adenovirus infection in *Neophema* parakeets, the clinical signs can mimic paramyxovirus infection. Confirmation of diagnosis is by histopathology, principally of the liver but also kidney and pancreas, and various laboratory tests.
• Chlamydia infection does not often cause CNS signs. Check by laboratory ELISA (inhibitory ELISA; i.e., BELISA) test.
• Poisoning is also another possibility.

(b) Treatment of this flock would consist of antibiotics (after sensitivity testing) for a minimum of 10 days. Some birds may be completely cured, others may remain carriers. Therefore control monitoring of all birds at the termination of therapy should be performed, with at least three negative cultures obtained over a period of 3 weeks before the flock can be considered *Salmonella* free. The premises must also be thoroughly cleaned and disinfected.

67 (a) The two eggs were laid by different individuals. The domesticated farmed ostrich is derived from at least three of the original subspecies that came from slightly different habitats (e.g., the blue-necked South African ostrich, the red-necked North African ostrich, and the now extinct Syrian ostrich of the Arabian deserts).
(b) The eggs of the different subspecies were not all exactly the same. There is also a lesser variation within the different subspecies. The genotype of the farmed ostrich is variable and is a mixture of the different subspecies. This variation in shell quality and texture is important in commercial practice because the different shells lose water at different rates and so will need incubation at slightly different relative humidities (i.e., the eggs must be sorted into batches all with shells of similar texture).

68 (a) Failure of the crop to empty properly is due to crop stasis and may be indicative of an overall stasis of the whole alimentary canal. There are numerous causes, including the following:
• Food of unsuitable consistency, food that is too cold, or food that is too hot and causes crop burns and stasis.
• Foreign bodies in the crop or anywhere in the gastrointestinal tract. This obstruction can be caused by bedding material or fibrous food (e.g., raw carrot, apple).
• Infection is either localized in the crop (e.g., *Candida*) or systemic (e.g., polyomavirus, any of the Enterobacteriaceae).
Failure of the crop to empty properly leads to overstretching and atony. This results in solidification of the retained food, fermentation (sour crop), and infection.
(b) Treatment consists of gentle flushing with warmed normal saline using a gavage tube and if necessary very careful massage to break up any concretions. Give subcutaneous or interosseous fluids. If crop infection is suspected, use nystatin and a broad-spectrum antibiotic (e.g., oral doxycycline or cephalosporins, but not fluoroquinolones or sulphur drugs, which may cause joint cartilage or feather defects in growing birds because of possible dehydration in these cases. A pendulous crop that does not retract can be supported with a "bra" made of self-adhesive elastic bandage. Feed less volume and a more liquid diet and feed more frequently.

69 (a) Self-mutilation resulting in chewing and plucking of the feathers that sometimes progresses to self-trauma to the skin is a common psychosis of psittacine birds. Gray parrots have the highest incidence, but the syndrome is also seen in many other psittacine birds, including conures, Amazon parrots, macaws, and even budgerigars.
(b) All of these species normally live in flocks, where there is a constant behavioral interaction and stimulation between other members of the flock. Isolated, single birds often confined in a small cage suffer boredom, lack of stimulation, and lack of attention when left by their owners for prolonged periods. Alternatively, excessive attention or overstimulation by children, being shouted at, or the introduction of a barking puppy can all precipitate the condition. A change in the bird's routine, alteration of the position of the bird's cage, redecoration of the room, or severe clipping of the wing feathers can all cause psychologic stress and start the bird self-mutilating.

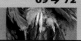

(c) Typically the first clinical signs are chewing of the ends of the contour feathers, usually as a result of excessive preening. This commences over the breast, with all the feathering eventually being damaged and lost. Next the flight feathers, including the tail, are attacked, so that only the crushed and split stumps remain. In the case of the "feather picker" the plumage on the head and upper neck is normal.

(d) Therapy is aimed at removing the initiating cause. Sometimes it is suspected that the lack of a mate may cause sexual frustration, in which case the bird's sex must first be determined by laparoscopy or by blood or feather DNA testing. If a mate is obtained, this bird must be introduced very carefully and *not* just placed in the same cage, which could result in it being attacked and even killed.

Some birds respond to the use of haloperidol and other human antipsychotic drugs. These may be given in the drinking water, with the dose gradually increased until the optimum dose for the particular bird is achieved and then maintained for several months. The use of an Elizabethan collar should only be considered as the absolute last resort. In some severely prolonged cases the feather follicles are so badly damaged that they never recover.

70 (a) This bird is a Harris' Hawk *(Parabuteo unicinctus).*

(b) The wing on the observer's left (i.e., the bird's right wing) is normal, whereas that on the other side cannot be extended to the same degree because of the formation of the scar tissue in the propatagial membrane. Also, this has resulted in the proximal attachment of the leading edge of the wing being displaced slightly caudally. This has happened because of collision trauma and subsequent strapping of the wing to the body for a prolonged period of convalescence. This condition severely limits the bird's flying ability.

(c) Repair of this structure is difficult because of the pars elastica (i.e., the ligament of insertion of the *M. tensor propatagialis pars longus*), which, together with the complex web of elastic fibers supporting the propatagial membrane, forms the leading edge of the wing. Damage to this area will heal successfully only after meticulous surgical technique.

71 (a) Hyperthyroidism tends to induce molting and increase the rate of feather growth. Hypothyroidism tends to produce obesity, reduced fertility, and a ragged, dull plumage together with symmetric feather loss without signs of pruritus. There is often decreased feather growth and feather abnormalities, such as a black discoloration of the feather tips. For hyperplasia of the thyroid gland see the answers to Figs. 36 and 37.

(b) Standard laboratory tests for thyroid dysplasia in birds are not well documented, but it is possible to carry out a plasma T_4 thyroxin estimation both before and 32 hours after administration of thyroid stimulating hormone or, if this is not available, thyroid releasing hormone (15 µg/kg). There should be a two- to fivefold increase in the level of plasma T_4 thyroxin if the gland is functional.

(c) In most cases, dark discoloration of the feathers is not due to thyroid disease but to a chronic hepatosis. In the case of this *Pionus* parrot the liver dysfunction accompanied by dyspnea was the result of a chronic aspergillosis of the lower respiratory tract and secondary to liver insufficiency. This was diagnosed after the evaluation of blood liver enzyme levels, microbiologic culture of a tracheal swab, and whole-body radiography.

72 (a) In birds, subcutaneous swellings may be caused by rupture of an air sac, but this is very unlikely to be the cause of swelling in this region. Ruptured air sacs or blocked air sac openings are usually associated with the proximal abdomen and thorax or the neck region. In birds, subcutaneous edema can result from bacterial infection or, rarely, iatrogenic drug overdosage.

(b) The massive subcutaneous edema with accompanying hyperemia and a bluish discoloration of the skin was caused by a generalized *Pseudomonas* infection. Diagnosis was confirmed using laboratory examination of skin and choanal and cloacal swabs.

(c) In raptors, wing tip edema is believed to be due to the bird being tethered to a perch (usually a block perch) during cold, frosty weather when the ground temperature and the adjacent air temperature is below freezing.

73 (a) There is sudden apathy, anorexia, loss of voice, and often dyspnea. Shocked birds usually sit on the floor of the cage with closed eyes and ruffled feathers in an effort to conserve body heat. Sometimes pale mucous membranes can be seen.

(b) Treatment consists of avoiding stress so far as is practical and placing the bird in a warm (26° to 30° C [79° to 86° F]) and quiet environment with subdued lighting. In birds the size of a budgerigar a bolus of 1 mL warm intravenous fluid (at body temperature) should be administered via the jugular vein. Fluid such as lactated Ringer's (Hartmann's) solution should be given. In larger birds, fluid therapy can be administered using the interosseous route into the ulna or tibia. If respiratory distress is evident, oxygen therapy should be instituted. Some clinicians advocate the use of corticosteroids but nonsteroidal antiinflammatory drugs are probably better.

74 (a) This lesion is probably caused by the protozoan parasite *Trichomonas*, which can infect all species of birds and cause lesions anywhere in the gastrointestinal tract or respiratory system. Gross lesions of this parasite can easily be mistaken for those of candidiasis. Differential diagnosis should also include *Avipoxvirus* infection, capillariasis, pigeon herpesvirus infection, and mycoplasmosis. Infection arises from contaminated food and water and from adult pigeons feeding youngsters. Clinically unaffected carrier birds probably maintain the infection.

(b) Dimetridazole or metronidazole (for oral administration to individual birds) combined with broad-spectrum antibiotics are used to treat possible secondary infections. However, resistance to the "azole" drugs is widespread because of misuse of these drugs by pigeon keepers. Vitamin A should also be administered parentally.

75 (a) This abnormality of the cere is termed *brown hypertrophy*. It is the result of excessive cornification of the cere with the keratin building up in layers. It is not uncommon in older female birds and may be influenced by estrogen levels.

(b) In the female bird it is of no clinical significance unless the accumulation of keratin blocks the nares. In male birds this condition may be an indication of gonadal neoplasm.

(c) The hypertrophic keratin can be removed by first softening it with a bland cream or olive oil and then carefully paring it away with a knife or forceps.

76 Some known toxins can cause feather disorders, especially during molting. Iatrogenic feather dystrophies have been frequently observed but have not been well documented, particularly regarding the histopathology. Delayed feather growth, feather defects, and other disorders are seen, especially in young pigeons, after the use of fluoroquinolones, fenbendazole, and various drugs for the treatment of coccidiosis, if these are administered during the molt. In young, unfeathered birds, chlortetracycline can also result in feather dystrophy. These abnormalities usually disappear after the next molt.

77 (a) The abnormal coloration and bar marking of some feathers (i.e., green to red) and the nonuniform growth of the plumage indicates the bird had periods of mineral deficiency that may have been related to egg laying. Chronic egg laying, gross obesity, and various other factors may result in a deficiency of calcium, phosphorus, and other minerals that influence metabolic pathways. Apart from alterations in color, the plumage of birds with mineral deficiencies is dull, lacks sheen, and is fragile. In these conditions, symmetric feather loss, molting disorders, and discoloration are common.

(b) Regarding therapy, measures should be taken to reduce chronic egg laying (e.g., decrease the period of daylight stimulation, reduce the caloric intake of the diet, remove the male bird and nest box). Hormone therapy, such as medroxyprogesterone acetate (25 mg/kg), can be used. The diet should be adjusted so that there is adequate mineral and vitamin D_3 intake and a balanced calcium to phosphorous ratio.

78 (a) This lesion was caused by frostbite. These birds are not well adapted to cold climates. In cold weather, when perches and wire netting are covered in frost, the birds hang onto these, causing the ice to partially melt and then refreeze, so that the bird becomes stuck to the frozen perch. The claws can be amputated as the bird tries to free itself.

(b) These birds should be provided with an enclosed and heated bird room attached to the outside aviary. They are best confined inside during frosty or inclement weather. Frostbite can occur in other species of birds, particularly tropical species such as tropical waterfowl and flamingoes.

79 First, a systematic examination, including radiography, clinical profile, and parasitology, should be performed. Apart from the assessment of any fractures and the chances of these healing so that there would be no permanent flying disability, it is essential to take into account any trauma to the soft tissues (e.g., muscle, nerve, propatagium) and to try to determine why the bird became a casualty in the first place. Was this bird at risk because it was already ill or weak from another complicating factor (e.g., parasites, mycobacteriosis)? Was the bird found in the wrong type of habitat for the time of year because it had recently been released by an ill-informed but well-meaning rescuer? Could recent stormy weather have blown the bird into an obstruction or electric wire? Was the bird shot or attacked by a predator but managed to escape and hide? A thorough assessment of the situation is essential to prevent the bird suffering further injury.

80 (a) Granulomatous dermatitis is often due to an infection with mycobacteria. In these lesions the skin becomes thickened with the accumulation of large macrophages in the dermis and subcutis. On histopathologic examination the macrophages are seen to contain numerous acid-fast–staining tubercle bacilli. Alternatively, chronic nontuberculous bacterial dermatitis can also result in granuloma formation. In this case this was due to an infection with *Escherichia coli*. Often this type of granuloma is composed of single or multiple nodules. Neoplasms can also produce granulomatous-like lesions.

(b) For a definitive diagnosis, surgical removal of the mass and histopathologic examination are necessary. Over the skull the skin is often tight and adherent to the underlying bone. If there is a difficulty closing the gap left after surgical removal of such a lesion, skin can often be mobilized from the proximal neck area.

81 Beak injuries of this sort are most commonly caused by bite wounds from cage mates and often occur during the breeding season, even amongst previously compatible pairs. Usually it is the male bird that attacks the hen. He may continue to do this even when placed with another hen, making him unfit to be paired.

Both the horny keratin and the underlying bone of the mandible may be fractured.

149

Aside from the systemic use of antibiotics such as clindamycin (10 mg/kg q8-12h), wiring the two halves of the beak together and overlaying this with a medical acrylic (as used for the repair of human dentures) or other suitable cyanoacrylate preparation produces acceptable resolution.

82 **(a)** Canary finches *(Serinus canaria)*, particularly if inbred, can sometimes produce genetic feather dystrophies. These defects may be seen as a curling and rolling of some of the long contour feathers. Some feathers may be retained in their sheaths, and others may be surrounded by a fibrous capsule so as to form a feather cyst, which may contain the cheese-textured remains of one or more feathers. These cysts may be dispersed over the whole body and appear as multiple hard, yellow accumulations or lumps of keratin.
(b) These signs are seen most often in Norwich canaries (a specific breed of *S. canaria*).
(c) Feather cysts are also seen in some psittacine species, particularly macaws but also in budgerigars and *Pionus* parrots, and are usually located on the wing. The only wild species in which feather cysts have been documented is the wild turkey.
(d) Feather cysts and deformed feathers can be surgically removed. However, excision requires very careful dissection to avoid distortion of the neighboring feather follicles. Otherwise, the feathers emerging from these can also become distorted and form cysts. Complete resolution of this condition is difficult.

83 A normally developed egg is present in the caudal abdominal region. From the radiograph it is not possible to determine the exact site of the egg within the oviduct or whether it is actually within the oviduct or free in the abdominal cavity. An indistinct soft tissue mass is noticeable dorsal to the egg. This could be an egg without a shell or part of the intestinal tract. An increase in radiodensity can be seen in both humeri, coracoids, femurs, and tibiotarsal bones. This is called *medullary bone* and is a normal physiologic feature of female birds in the egg-laying phase and is influenced by estrogens. Medullary bone functions as a calcium store that can be mobilized for the laying down of calcium in the egg shell during its passage through the shell gland.

84 Radiodense heavy metal particles are visible in the cloaca. The bird's primary disease may therefore have been heavy metal intoxication. Nonabsorbable contrast agent is visible in both lungs and part of the air sacs, indicating the bird has aspirated a large amount of barium sulfate.
General radiographic principles, such as the preparation of a plain radiograph before the use of a contrast agent, are also important in birds, for example, to avoid overseeing any heavy metal particles as a result of the superimposition of the contrast medium. However, before proceeding with contrast radiography the patient should be fasted for about 2 hours to prevent regurgitation. Because of this risk, some authorities advise against the use of anesthesia. Inhalation of the comparatively large barium sulfate particles can cause a tissue reaction in the lung and associated dyspnea. However, this is rarely seen in birds, even when large quantities of barium sulfate are aspirated, as in the case illustrated.

85 **(a)** This family of birds, Capitonidae, are tropical birds that are strongly built and have big heads, stout bills, and short legs. They are related to toucans and woodpeckers. Capitonidae feed on fruit, berries, buds, some insects, and, in the case of the larger species, lizards, mice, and smaller birds.
(b) Examination of the bird consisted of visual and palpable examination of the foot and the unfeathered short legs and manipulation of all the joints. This revealed a slight swelling

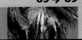

and stiffness of the stifle joint. Radiography demonstrated a lesion involving the distal end of the femur. There was some osteolysis, some remodeling of the cortex, and soft tissue swelling. After euthanasia, histopathology indicated an osteosarcoma.

86 (a) Various infectious agents should be considered in your differential diagnoses, such as *Paramyxovirus* type 4 infection, reovirus (orthovirus) infection, mycobacteriosis, aspergillosis, *Chlamydia* infection, toxoplasmosis, and possibly filariasis. Possible noninfectious etiologies include lead and zinc toxicity, aflatoxins, and exotic household plants. Head trauma or a neoplasm might be considered. If there is a history of episodic seizure with polydipsia or polyuria, consider a hypothalamic or pituitary tumor. After a detailed anamnesis (e.g., whether this is the only bird affected, which would indicate a noninfectious etiology or aspergillosis), thorough clinical examination (looking for signs of trauma, particularly from a cage mate), and radiographic examination (especially for lead particles in the gastrointestinal tract), laboratory tests for infectious agents should be performed before a definitive diagnosis is reached.
(b) Symptomatic therapy may help to stabilize the bird. This should include the use of electrolytes (if a head trauma has been ruled out). Use of B vitamins (especially if endoparasites are suspected) may help. The bird should be kept in a warm, quiet environment with subdued lighting.

87 (a) During the course of psittacine beak and feather disease (see Figs. 22, 47, and 48), beak and nail deformities often ultimately develop. The beak can become elongated, malformed, and necrotic, and fault lines can occur. The beak may be excessively shiny as a result of the lack of the production of powder down (compare with Fig. 22). A dystrophy of the beak in psittacine beak and feather disease can lead to an inability to eat seed.
(b) A malformed beak can result from various causes, such as trauma or improper incubation, or it can occur in malnourished birds, such as those suffering from metabolic bone disease. The final diagnosis of this condition is described in the answer to Figs. 47 and 48.

88 (a) The propatagial membrane is the elasticated part of the wing filling in the triangular area between the humerus and the radius. It forms the leading edge of the wing between the shoulder and the radiocarpal joint.
(b) The illustration shows this area to be affected with a exudative dermatitis accompanied by some feather loss. A lesion of this sort is often accompanied by a marked pruritus, resulting in automutilation, secondary infection, and possible death.
(c) Staphylococci are the most common microorganisms involved in avian skin infections, but various other bacteria such as *Escherichia coli*, *Clostridia*, and *Pseudomonas* organisms can also cause feather disorders and dermatitis. Skin lesions often arise from mechanical damage, such as feather picking or being attacked by a cage mate or predator. In some longstanding cases, chronic, nontuberculous bacterial dermatitis can also lead to granuloma formation. The granuloma may be solitary or multiple, and the lesions are usually nodular.
(d) To differentiate this type of lesion from a neoplasm, histopathology and microbiologic culture must be performed.

89 (a) Protection of the radiographer is most important; therefore lead gloves should be worn. The hands should be kept out of the primary beam, which should be coned down to the minimum necessary to cover the area being radiographed. Because it is difficult to hold a budgerigar when the hands are protected by lead gloves, it may be necessary to protect the hands by an overlaid leaded rubber sheet. The table should be covered with a lead sheet to minimize scatter and the penetration of the primary beam to floor level.

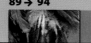

(b) If possible, other methods of positioning the bird should be used, such as a custom-made restraint board with a sheet made of Perspex or thick (0.5 cm or less), rigid polythene. Alternatively, the bird can be deeply sedated with diazepam or lightly anaesthetized, preferably with isoflurane, which is probably less stressful for the bird. For quality radiographs, correct positioning with an absolutely still subject is essential.

90 The lungs show nonuniform increases in radiodensity with thickening of the caudal thoracic air sac. This bird was suffering from a chronic infection of the respiratory tract.
This bird had aspergillosis, which could be confirmed by serology. Infertility is quite common in these birds because of the effects of mycotoxins on the gonads.

91 (a) The common contrast media used in birds are positive-contrast media (barium sulphate and organic iodine compounds) and negative-contrast media (air).
(b) The most commonly used contrast medium is nonabsorbable barium sulfate, which is used to demonstrate the gastrointestinal tract. The dosage is 20 ml/kg, administered by cannula or gavage tube directly into the crop. Gastrointestinal transit time varies depending on the species and the normal type of diet consumed by the bird (i.e., frugivorous, graniverous, carnivorous, etc.). Double-contrast studies of the gastrointestinal tract can be achieved using air or barium sulfate orally or into the cloaca and rectum. These radiographic techniques are indicated if lesions of the gastrointestinal mucosa are suspected. For urography, birds need sedation or light anesthesia. The organic iodine compound is administered intravenously after having been warmed to body temperature. Radiography is carried out at 30 seconds and 1 minute after injection and will demonstrate the kidney and ureters.

92 (a) Elongated and twisted claws are often seen in old canaries and some other captive passeriformes. No definitive etiology has been documented for these malformed claws, although it has been suggested that hepatopathy, inbreeding, and unsuitable perches may be contributing factors. This bird also shows the beginnings of hyperkeratinization, and there is an emerging pododermatitis ("bumblefoot") lesion.
(b) The bird's claws should be trimmed regularly and the bird kept on cloth-covered perches soaked in povidone-iodine solution or chlorhexidine. Attention should be paid to improving the diet. Scrupulous cage hygiene should be observed.

93 (a) The left leg is not hanging limply but is held with the foot in a cramped position. This indicates the leg is probably not broken but rather is in spasm, and some or all of the tissues in the leg could be inflamed. This could indicate a neuritis, possible pressure on the nerves of this leg from a neoplasm of the left kidney or gonad, a unilateral nephritis, or possible egg binding.
(b) Radiography of the whole body, in both dorsoventral and lateral projections, should be the first investigation performed, followed by a complete clinical profile, which may indicate a leukocytosis and, rarely, a raised plasma uric acid. It is also possible to obtain biopsy samples from the kidney under direct vision using an endoscope while performing an endoscopic examination of the kidney and adjacent tissues. Ultrasonography is also a useful diagnostic aid.

94 (a) There is a prominent papilloma-like growth involving the rostral commissure of the rima glottis.
(b) These neoplasms are sometimes associated with the papillomavirus and in psittaciformes are not uncommonly found in the oropharynx, the upper gastrointestinal tract, and the cloaca.

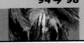

(c) Diagnosis can be confirmed by biopsy. Use a radiosurgical instrument to very carefully remove a piece of tissue. Follow with cauterization with a silver nitrate pencil and controlling the action of this with saline solution.

(d) Any bleeding during surgery will help to stimulate autoimmune response. An autogenous vaccine can also be prepared from the harvested tissue.

95 **(a)** The not uncommon abnormal change in coloration of the cere of male budgerigars (from blue to brown) is sometimes associated with neoplasia of the testes. If this discoloration were the only clinical sign, the cause could be any hormonal imbalance.

(b) A radiograph and/or an ultrasonographic examination might help to diagnose the soft tissue lesion and the tumorous nature of the mass. The use of a barium contrast may show the intestine displaced from its normal position by the neoplasm. Diagnostic laparotomy or biopsy may be indicated in a few cases.

96 The caudal lung border appears more rounded than normal. This is seen as a nonspecific sign of mild lung disease. Birds do not usually exhibit clinical symptoms of respiratory tract disease at this stage.

This bird also has a large amount of grit in the ventriculus (gizzard), which may be a sign of gastrointestinal malfunction.

97 **(a)** This is a rhinolith, or collection of necrotic debris resulting in a proliferative granulomatous lesion.

(b) This is the end result of a persistent rhinitis, which is part of a prolonged upper respiratory disease resulting from hypovitaminosis A and some environmental irritants, included in which are cigarette smoke, excessive powder down (of in-contact cockatiels or cockatoos), and dust from dried bedding or floor covering. Other possible irritants are household aerosols and diesel fumes from a nearby highway. These birds normally inhabit humid, tropical rainforests, and the excessively dry atmosphere of a centrally heated house may predispose to this condition. Secondarily these lesions become infected with a variety of microorganisms. In this particular case it was predominantly *Klebsiella* sp.

(c) This necrotic debris should be very carefully removed. The area is quite vascular, and bleeding easily occurs, resulting in the area filling with blood clot. After the debris is removed, the area requires microbiologic evaluation, daily cleaning with providone-iodine solution, chlorhexidine, or proflavine cream, and application of appropriate antibiotics. Bad cases can result in atrophic rhinitis with a patent opening between the two nostrils. Some veterinarians suggest using a human dental preparation as a substitute for hydrophilic dressing, to encourage epithelization.

There is some evidence that damage to some of the inner nostril structures can result in immunosuppression.

98 **(a)** Renal disease can lead to feather loss without significant pruritus, feather dystrophies, or associated dermatitis. Chronic renal disease often results in feather loss over the thorax and abdomen, along with abnormal dominance of semiplumes instead of the normal contour feathers.

(b) The appearance of this condition in its advanced stages should be differentiated from psittacine beak and feather disease (exhibiting extensive hyperkeratosis, feather loss and feather malformation, and associated dermatitis), which is caused by a circovirus.

(c) Prognosis in these cases is usually poor. Dietary measures, as well as antibiotic therapy in proven bacterial etiologies, could be helpful.

99 (a) This illustration shows gross enlargement of the parathyroid glands, indicating a secondary nutritional hyperparathyroidism.
(b) This results from a diet deficient in calcium. The diet of captive parrots is often composed almost entirely of sunflower seed. This bird also had metabolic bone disease, which was revealed by radiography.

100 (a) This bird has mucopurulent blepharitis and conjunctivitis with associated abscess formation at the nasal canthus and prolapse of the nictitating membrane.
(b) Lesions of the eyelids are commonly caused by traumatic injuries such as bites. These may result in superficial or perforating wounds. Such injuries are frequently followed by secondary bacterial infection resulting in a mucopurulent exudate and abscess formation. Prolapse of the nictitating membrane can occur in cases of toxicity (e.g., botulism), trauma (as described above), or infectious disease (e.g., *Paramyxovirus* infection).
(c) If the prolapse persists after treating the secondary bacterial infection, partial surgical removal of some of the third eyelid may be necessary. However, total removal is unwise because it may result in xerophthalmia.

101 Disturbances of the intraocular pressure resulting in glaucoma are rare in birds. Primary glaucoma has not as yet been documented in birds. Secondary glaucoma may occur in the course of an infection and after luxation of the lens into the anterior chamber.
Clinical signs are sensitivity to light, irritation, enlargement of the bulb, reddening and swelling of other parts of the eye, a dilated pupil, and limited visual activity.
In this particular case glaucoma occurred subsequent to trauma.

102 (a) The parasite illustrated is *Sternostoma trachaecolum,* commonly known as the "air sac mite." These parasites are found throughout the respiratory system in many *Passeriforme* species, especially finches, such as canaries *(Serinus canaria)* and Gouldian finches *(Chloebia gouldiae).*
(b) The life cycle is apparently direct, with transmission between adults by contaminated food and adult birds infecting nestlings when feeding them. Other species of *Sternostoma* occur in passeriformes, as does the less common respiratory mite *Cytodites nudus,* which also occurs in some galliformes.
(c) Clinical signs include wheezing, loss of voice, in some cases a characteristic clicking during respiration, dyspnea, and open-mouth breathing. However, subclinical infection is common.
Parasites located in the trachea may be visualized as small dark specks by transillumination of the trachea after wetting the feathers of the neck with a little alcohol. Otherwise autopsy is the only way to establish a diagnosis. Infection with this parasite is sometimes complicated by secondary infection.
(d) Treatment is by topical application to the skin on the dorsum of the neck or thorax of one drop of ivermectin 1%. Alternatively, a dichlorvos strip may be applied, but this should be used strictly according to the manufacturer's instructions.

103 (a) Egg-bound birds are often shocked. They sit fluffed up on the bottom of the cage, often in respiratory distress, and may appear to be straining. Sometimes the vent is pasted and swollen. Often the egg can be palpated through the abdominal wall or seen through the vent. The bird may have laid several eggs and then stopped. Occasionally an old captive household parrot (e.g., 30 years of age) that has never laid an egg before suddenly becomes egg-bound with a single egg.

(b) In the radiograph an abnormally small egg with a hypocalcified shell can be seen in the caudal abdominal region. Hypocalcification of the egg in pet birds usually indicates that the egg has remained in the shell gland (or calcium-producing region of the oviduct) for a long period, probably because the bird is not entirely physically fit. An indistinct soft tissue mass is also visible, displacing the grit-filled ventriculus dorsally (i.e., above the imaginary horizontal line between the two hips) and to the left. With ultrasonography this mass was seen to be three laminated eggs. The bird was treated surgically, with all the eggs removed via salpingotomy. Medullary bone formation can be seen in the radius, ulna, femur, and tibiotarsal bones.

(c) Normally, egg-bound birds can be treated with injections of calcium borogluconate (10%, or 100 mg/ml) at a dose of 50 mg/kg body weight by *slow* intravenous injection, along with oxytocin (10 IU/ml 0.3 to 0.5 ml/kg body weight). Alternatively, dinoprost (5 mg/ml), a prostaglandin, can be used at a dose of 0.02 to 0.1 mg/kg body weight once only. Keeping the bird on a warm pad helps to alleviate shock and relax the vent. Also keep the bird in a calm and warm environment and apply paraffin oil to the cloaca.

104 (a) There is an overall lack of density in the cortex of all the limb bones. Both tibiotarsal bones show a proximal varus of the diaphysis. The ulna on the right side shows signs of healing fracture. The soft tissue shadow of the abdominal viscera is greatly enlarged, which may or may not be physiologic in a nestling of this age because of an increase in body fat.

(b) This bird is suffering from metabolic bone disease. This a common occurrence in artificially reared parrots that do not receive the correct balance of amount of calcium and phosphorus or adequate vitamin D_3 in their diet. It is also documented as occurring in both artificially reared and wild raptors, in wild vultures, and in pigeons.

105 (a) This bird suffers from a disease called *perosis*. A primary or secondary lack of manganese, caused by an excess of calcium, and a deficiency of choline in the diet are considered responsible for this disease. Affected birds show thickened hocks together with bending deformities of the tibiotarsus and tarsometatarsus, resulting in luxation of the Achilles tendon. This causes rotation of the intertarsal joint (up to 180 degrees) and prevents the normal use of the affected limb. Analogous clinical signs are caused by a lack of biotin and zinc. Perosis and perosis-like conditions are seen in galliformes (particularly when intensively reared), in waterfowl, and in ratites.

(b) Those species in which the young are fast growing when reared commercially are predisposed to the condition.

(c) The primary differential diagnosis is metabolic bone disease in which the stability of the joints is normal but mineralization of the bone is affected (see the answer to Fig. 104). This can be checked by radiography.

(d) In the early stages of perosis, successful surgical reduction of the Achilles tendon luxation can be achieved by suturing the tendon sheath to the retinaculum and periosteum over the lateral aspect of the trochlear.

106 (a) The organisms seen are colonies of *Candida* spp. In Gram's stain, they appear like gram-positive bacteria but can easily be differentiated from these by their larger size compared with bacteria and by the occurrence of budding.

(b) *Candida* organisms form part of the autochthonous flora of birds and can often be isolated in smaller amounts without having any pathologic effects on affected tissue. Pathogenicity should be considered if *Candida* is the dominant microorganism on culture or if other findings or symptoms indicate *Candida* is involved in the disease process. Such diseases often occur after the following:

- Prolonged antibiotic therapy
- Immunosuppressed birds (excessively stressed or after the use of corticosteroids)
- The integrity of the skin or mucosa is impaired (burns, trauma, hypovitaminosis A, etc.).

Young birds with an immature immune system are especially prone to candidiasis, and such disease is most common in the gastrointestinal tract and the skin.

107 External splinting of a fracture of the tibiotarsal bone in a raptor, particularly using plaster of paris, is not suitable. The plaster of paris is too heavy for a relatively lightweight creature. It is difficult to achieve good stability of the fractured segments of the bone because of the shape of the leg, which is rather like an elongated cone. In the case illustrated the cast looks quite loose at the proximal end and is bearing awkwardly on the foot, which looks swollen. There is no sign of padding material beneath the plaster.

Although the bird has placed its foot on the perch and the leg looks straight, it would be surprising if this cast resulted in a completely satisfactory result. In most cases use must be made of a variety of internal splinting techniques using stainless steel pins but always reinforced by an external splint of material such as Hexcelite or an aluminum finger splint.

108 **(a)** A trypanosome is located at approximately 7 o'clock in the illustration. At approximately 2 o'clock in the illustration is an intracytoplasmic *Plasmodium* organism, or avian malarial parasite.

(b) Trypanosomes are found in a variety of different types of birds, among which are passeriformes, galliformes, anseriformes, columbiformes, and raptors. The parasites are transmitted by biting arthropods, including louse flies (hippoboscids) and red mites (*Dermanyssus* spp.). Trypanosomes apparently do not cause disease in birds.

(c) Avian malarial parasites can be seen to have typically occupied approximately 25% to 40% of the cytoplasm and to have slightly displaced the nucleus. There are at least 25 species of avian malarial parasite transmitted by various species of mosquito. The parasites infect a wide variety of birds and may or may not be pathogenic. Many wild passeriformes may act as latent carriers of the *Plasmodium* organism. When causing disease (e.g., in pigeons, waterfowl, penguins, and some raptors) there is a hemolytic anemia leading to black discolored hepatosplenomegaly and bright green feces (increased biliverdin). Dyspnea, vomiting, and subcutaneous hemorrhage also occur.

109 **(a)** A chemosis is a swelling and congestion of the conjunctiva. This may be due to an inflammation of the conjunctiva resulting in edema or caused by circulatory problems. Excessive secretion and abnormal blood-filled tissue is commonly seen.

(b) *Chlamydia psittaci* was isolated from this chronic lesion and was the primary causal agent.

Although with chlamydiosis the clinical signs of a conjunctivitis are often prominent, the clinical picture may vary widely and may not always exhibit typical signs. Quite often the lesion may be complicated by secondary infection, consequently a laboratory examination specifically for *Chlamydia psittaci* and other microbiologic pathogens may be indicated in those cases of inflammatory eye disease that do not respond to routine treatment.

110 **(a)** Fluorescein staining can be used to demonstrate corneal wounds, as in mammals. The prognosis even in penetrating wounds, if they are *not* infected, is always good because of excellent corneal regeneration. Corneal wounds usually heal rapidly with an occasional small scar and a focal pigmentation seen on the surface.

(b) Systemic and local topical antibiotic therapy should be applied. If necessary a tarsorrhaphy can be carried out and the sutures left in place for several days. Use injectable vitamin A.

(c) Corneal defects may be complicated by secondary infection leading to abscess formation and a reduced visual acuity. In the case of keratitis, mucopurulent exudation and ulceration commonly occur as a result of bacterial infection. A more viscous discharge with corneal ulceration may be seen as a result of mycotic infection, such as *Candida* spp. One complication of a corneal defect is ulceration.

111 In the normal bird it is not possible to visualize the kidneys sonographically by transcutaneous ultrasonography. Demonstration of this organ in this particular case by ultrasound indicates a pathologic process. The outlines of the abnormal kidney can be clearly identified, and inhomogeneous structures are visible in the parenchyma. Three well-defined anechoic areas (fluid, which can be classified as cysts) and areas of hyperechogenicity are visible in the renal parenchyma. Together, these findings indicate a neoplastic change of the kidney. Because of its position close to the ischiadic nerve, enlargement of this organ is often seen in combination with paresis or paralysis of the legs.

112 The contour of the oviduct can easily be recognized. Within this organ there are four larger and several smaller round areas, all of which are surrounded by structures of inhomogeneous density. Of the four larger formations, two show a texture of nonhomogenous echogenicity and the other two are characterized by hypoechoic areas. This ultrasonographic picture indicates the appearance of an oviduct containing several laminated eggs. During surgery, four of these eggs were removed, and in two cases there were signs of lysis within the centre of the egg. This example illustrates that laminated eggs and soft-shelled eggs can be identified with ultrasonography, whereas such a diagnosis cannot be established using radiographic imaging, as seen in Fig. 103.

113 The bird has an obvious fracture of the humerus on the left side of the illustration, with marked displacement of the fractured ends of the bone. There is an increased homogeneous increase in radiodensity of the lungs and air sac regions. This may be indicative of pneumonia/air sacculitis, which may be due to bacterial infection of the respiratory tract and is consistent with the dyspnea. In the case of open fractures of the pneumatized avian bones, such as the humerus, infection can be spread via the air sac system. A more uniform increase in radiodensity tends to indicate a bacterial infection, whereas a more inhomogeneous pattern is more commonly present in mycotic infections. However, this is not pathognomonic, and laboratory examination (e.g., tracheal microbiologic swabs) must be used to make a definitive diagnosis.

114 Differential diagnoses include the following:
- *Atoxoplasma* sp. This is quite pathogenic, often showing few clinical signs.
- Other cyst-forming protozoans, such as *Eimeria* spp., *Isospora* spp., or *Dorisiella* spp., which are less pathogenic than *Atoxoplasma* infection. These organisms often produce blood-stained feces.
- Nematode infection, particularly *Ascaridia* spp. or *Capillaria* spp. Both of these can build up in intensively stocked aviaries.
- *Plasmodium* spp. or *Leucocytozoon* spp., but only if the weather conditions are right for the transmitting biting insects.
- Enterobacteriaceae, such as *Salmonella* spp. and *Escherichia coli*. These bacterial diseases are usually not chronic wasting diseases, and they often produce dysphagia and enteritis.

157

• Both *Mycobacterium* and *Megabacterium* infections produce chronic wasting diseases but are not usually epizootic.
• Candidiasis should be considered, but this usually results in dysphagia.
• *Dermanyssus* and *Ornithonyssus* organisms can produce chronic wasting disease with severe anemia.
A generalized hyperemia of the exterior of the carcass occurs, which may be due to an acute inflammatory reaction in response to a secondary infection.

115 **(a)** It looks as though this young bird is begging for food from its handler, in which case it has almost certainly become imprinted on this person.
(b) Birds that are imprinted on their human handlers become totally dependent on them. Such birds do not recognize their own species, may not recognize their normal range of prey species, and probably will not be capable of hunting for their normal prey. They are extremely difficult to release back into the wild effectively and may even become a danger to unsuspecting persons whom the bird may "attack," believing them to be a ready source of food.

116 As in the case of this pigeon, periocular swelling is more commonly seen during the course of disease affecting the nose, infraorbital sinus, and entire upper respiratory tract rather than as a result of primary ocular disease. Microbiologic infections of the upper respiratory tract are often associated with mucus or purulent secretion of the eye. The formation of purulent material within the paraorbital sinuses may look similar to an exophthalmus and can lead to misinterpretation.

117 The three volatile aesthetics most commonly used for avian anesthesia are halothane, methoxyflurane, and isoflurane. In the past both ether and cyclopropane have been used successfully. However, both are highly explosive, and ether is very irritating to respiratory epithelium.
Without doubt, at present isoflurane is the anesthetic of choice for birds. It provides rapid induction and recovery times, as well as low organ toxicity, and consequently has the highest margin of safety. Muscle relaxation is excellent during the anesthetic stage used for surgery. Because of isoflurane's low blood solubility, the depth of anesthesia can be regulated quickly and accurately. Should apnea occur as a result of overdosage, it happens well before the onset of cardiac arrest, allowing immediate effective counter-measures to be instituted. This considerably reduces the risk of death caused by the anesthetic.
Halothane is the most commonly used volatile anesthetic in general veterinary practice. However, compared with isoflurane, its safety margin is lower. Induction and recovery take longer and cardiopulmonary depression is more evident than with isoflurane. Also there is a potential for catecholamine sensitization and hepatotoxicity. If the patient is overdosed, cardiac and pulmonary arrest occur simultaneously.
Methoxyflurane is highly soluble in blood, which results in prolonged induction and recovery times. Muscle relaxation and analgesia are good. Cardiopulmonary depression and overdosage effects are similar to those of halothane. Methoxyflurane has a high potential for organ toxicity.

118 **(a)** Both constriction and dilator muscles have striated fibers. Movement of the pupil is to a large degree under voluntary control, and the pupillary light reflex is unreliable. The pupil responds poorly to light stimulation but actively to the bird's temperamental influence. There is no dilation of the pupil with atropine.

(b) The avian lens has a nonoptic ringlike peripheral region termed the *annular pad,* which is next to the ciliary processes. This region shows some interspecific variation, being well developed in diurnal birds of prey but reduced in diving and nocturnal birds.

Accommodation of the avian eye is very well developed. In some species this is because of the well-developed Crampton's muscle, the striated anterior sclerocorneal muscle, which is one of the two main ciliary muscles. This muscle pulls and distorts the cornea, thereby increasing its curvature and refractive index. However, in birds overall there is considerable interspecific variation in the different parts of the ciliary muscles and in the actual mechanism of accommodation, as well as in the softness of the avian lens, which is generally softer than in mammals.

119 (a) The color of the iris depends on age, gender, and species and can be black (e.g., adult male Moluccan cockatoo), brown (e.g., adult female Moluccan cockatoo), yellow, green, red, silvery gray, or pale blue. Because of this high degree of physiologic variation it can be difficult to give a judgment on abnormal coloration unless the observer is very familiar with a particular species.

(b) Discoloration of the iris together with atrophy may be seen after an iridocyclitis. In most cases this is irreversible, as in the gray parrot illustrated.

120 Although this cage is typical of many sold by the pet trade, it does not offer much scope for even limited flight exercise. The height is reasonable, but increasing the lateral length would improve the situation. The vertical bars and curved bars across the top of the cage the increase the risk of trapped wings. Horizontal cage bars would be better.

Perches made of plastic may be easily cleaned but offer no variety in diameter to exercise the feet and maintain healthy muscles and blood circulation. Instead, perches should be replaced by freshly cut branches of hardwood trees, such as fruit trees or beech *(Fagus sylvatica),* birch *(Betula* spp.), ash *(Fraxinus* spp.), or willow *(Salix* spp.) trees, which offer a variable diameter. Perches covered with sandpaper or a sandpaper sheet on the floor of the cage are abrasive to the pads of the feet and predispose to pododermatitis. The food and water containers should be placed high in the cage and covered (e.g., food containers attached outside the cage, with access ports through the bars). Column drink containers should be used. Loose seed on the floor of the cage should be discouraged. All of this is intended to prevent contamination of food and water with feces. Finally, the mirror should be replaced by a companion, but care should be taken with the introduction. In some species the established bird may resent and attack a new bird introduced into its own private space.

121 (a) These nematodes are gapeworms *(Syngamus trachea).*

(b) This parasite can probably infect all species of birds, and many wild passeriformes are infected. Ground-feeding birds are most commonly infected, but some raptors eat the transport hosts. Other similar nematodes infect waterfowl (e.g., *Cyathostoma bronchialis).*

(c) Adult male and female worms live in permanent union (Y-shaped) in the trachea. The double operculated, ellipsoidal eggs are coughed up into the oral cavity and then swallowed and excreted in the feces. The infectious larva take 8 to 14 days to develop within the egg. Infection occurs by ingestion of the embryonated egg or hatched larva or from a paratenic host (e.g., earthworms, snails, and various other invertebrates). The encysted larvae can survive for up to 4 years in earthworms, and the intake of contaminated transport hosts provides a higher risk to the bird because they may contain considerable numbers of infectious gapeworm encysted larvae. These larvae perforate the bird's intestines and pass via the bloodstream or directly via the visceral cavity to the lung, and from there they move to the trachea. Adult worms penetrate tracheal mucosa and suck blood, which results in the excessive production of mucous and produces symptoms such as gasping, coughing, wheezing, and head shaking. Mortality is low in adults but higher in young birds because of the smaller diameter of the trachea.

122 (a) This casting contains beetle wing castings and other indigestible pieces of the chitinous exoskeleton of insects. This tends to indicate the bird was not able to hunt effectively and was probably flightless.
(b) These castings are normal and would usually contain undigested structures of the prey (i.e., hair, feathers, bone, teeth, etc.).
If flightlessness is limited to wing problems, (e.g., a fracture) and there is little or no malaise, these birds will feed and maintain themselves on carrion, if they can find it, and on insects for some time. This depends on weather conditions, the bird's success in finding carrion, and on the bird's initial condition. Often the duration of flightlessness can be estimated by the degree of damage to the tail feathers, caused by their contact with the ground.

123 Severe dyspnea in birds is seen in diseases of the respiratory tract or with increased intraabdominal pressure from decreased respiratory volume resulting from compression of the thoracic and abdominal air sacs. This may be caused, for example, by organ enlargement or ascites. A *sudden* onset of severe respiratory distress is highly suspicious of obstruction of the upper respiratory airways by foreign bodies, usually inhaled food, or an aspergilloma that may have broken off and become wedged in the syrinx. Treatment consists of placing an air sac tube into the posterior thoracic air sac and insufflating this with oxygen. In upper respiratory obstructions, normal breathing will recommence almost immediately. As soon as the general condition of the bird has stabilized, anesthesia and endoscopic examination of the upper respiratory tract to remove the obstructing object can be carried out. Foreign bodies may be removed by aspiration or resection of the trachea.

124 (a) These radiodense structures in the kidneys are accumulations of uric acid crystals. They result from either the excessive production of uric acid (i.e., dietary protein imbalance in excess of bodily requirements), insufficient dilution of excessively high blood uric acid levels (resulting from severe and prolonged dehydration), or renal dysfunction (i.e., renal insufficiency caused by renal tubular disease or hypovitaminosis A, which influences mucopolysaccharide production and the vitality of epithelia).
(b) Renal uric acid depositions are indicators of nonspecific renal insufficiency and are often seen together with high blood levels of uric acid. However, they are not necessarily specific signs of gout. Raptors take up very little water and gain most of their fluid requirements from ingested food, as do many small xerophilic birds living in desert conditions. The presence of precipitated uric acid in the kidneys of a raptor might indicate a prolonged fasting or starvation period. However, further investigation, laboratory and otherwise, may be necessary to confirm the diagnosis. Also, some raptors, such as peregrine falcons *(Falco peregrinus),* have very high postprandial blood uric acid levels but do not develop uric acid crystal deposition.

125 (a) The radiograph shows small spots of increased radiodensity in the gastrointestinal tract that are ingested heavy metal particles and that are, in most cases, lead.
(b) This often occurs in psittacine birds because of their preference for chewing objects. Curtain weights; leaded windows; old metal toys; electricians' clips; old lead paint, usually in older houses; champagne and wine bottle foils; and costume jewelry are common sources for companion birds.

Symptoms depend on the amount ingested and the duration of lead intake. These symptoms include weakness, lethargy, anorexia, weight loss, regurgitation, diarrhea, abnormally colored feces, ataxia, and seizures.
Lead shot located in the muscles or subcutaneous tissue are usually encapsulated and do not cause any symptoms. Radiographic finding of lead shot in the muscles of a radiograph of an Amazon parrot has been reported.
To confirm the diagnosis and to monitor the effect of therapy, blood level testing is necessary. The absence of radiographic evidence does not eliminate lead intoxication.
(c) Treatment consists of the following measures:
• Removing all ingested heavy metal objects by gastric lavage using sodium sulfate with activated charcoal or liquid paraffin or via surgery.
• Chelation using sodium calcium edentate (10 to 40 mg/kg body weight IV or IM twice daily for at least 5 to 10 days) or dimercaprol BP (25 to 35 mg/kg PO or IM twice daily for 5 days, rest for 2 days, and repeat for 3 to 5 weeks).
• Seizures can usually be controlled by diazepam (0.5 to 1.5 mg/kg body weight IV or IM 3 times daily).
Fluid therapy may be necessary.

126 (a) Supraorbital and submandibular swellings are typical locations for squamous cell metaplasia caused by hypovitaminosis A. This condition produces circumscribed compact swellings around the lacrimal glands, respiratory sinuses, and salivary glands. In the oral cavity, squamous sell metaplasia is characterized by caseous white or yellow masses, especially in the perlingual region and around the choana.
(b) The owner should be asked about the bird's diet. Food that only consists of seeds and nuts is usually very low in vitamin A content. Even commercially available mixtures that contain vitamin A cannot be guaranteed because of a decrease in potency during unsuitable storage conditions.
(c) Treatment consists of resecting the caseous mass by incision and curettage. The diet should be adjusted by adding fruit and green vegetables or supplementing the drinking water with soluble vitamins. Short-term parental administration of vitamin A is advised (5000 IU/kg body weight q24h for 7 days).
(d) Hypovitaminosis A affects the vitality of all epithelial tissue, and therefore integrity of skin, respiratory system, urinogenital system, and alimentary canal may all be impaired and subject to microbiologic attack.

127 Luxations or even fractures of the cervical column in ratites are often related to restraint using an ostrich crook like a shepherd's crook. Ruptured blood vessels and other soft tissue damage are also associated problems.
An alternative method of catching and restraining ratites is to cover the head with a hood of dark cloth. A suitable hood can be made of the sleeve of a sweatshirt, held with the arm inside. When the bird's head or beak is grasped the sleeve is inverted over the bird's head and neck. Also, leading or herding birds into a darkened area, such as a building where the lights can be dimmed, or even catching the bird at night in total darkness with a small torch will also facilitate restraint. Tame individual birds can be controlled by guiding them in V-shaped restraining stocks or a crush with solid sides and a bar just below hip height to stop the bird reversing out and a strap to go over the shoulders. Any person involved in catching these large birds should be aware that ratites primarily defend themselves by kicking to chest height, and there is a high risk of injury for both man and bird (e.g., laceration of its own neck). Holding the bird's head down to within 18 inches of the ground tends to stop the bird kicking.

128 (a) This chick is approximately 14 days or slightly more in age. It has its second coat of down and is just acquiring its first plumage feathers. It will just be able to stand but will spend most of its time on its haunches.

(b) Regardless of the method this fledgling was acquired, the "owner" should be informed that it is illegal to take any bird from the wild and that that the bird must be legally registered and identified with a numbered ring or numbered cable tie issued by the appropriate government department wildlife division. The law may also require that the fledgling is reared by a suitably licensed person.

The chick is best kept at a temperature of 17° C (63° F). It is best confined in a vertical-sided cylindrical enclosure (about 8 inches high and 10 inches in diameter [250 mm high and 255 mm in diameter]) made of aluminum or plastic sheet so that it is easily cleaned. This bottomless cylinder is placed on newspaper, on top of which are layers of kitchen toweling or cotton towel to provide a nonslip, easily gripped surface that can be replenished when soiled. Hygiene is of paramount importance. Do not use wood shavings, sawdust, peat, or cat litter, all of which contaminate the food and cause crop impaction or respiratory problems.

(c) If the fledgling is to be released back into the wild, it must not become imprinted onto its human contacts and therefore must be fed by a glove puppet and out of human sight. The glove puppet should as nearly as possible resemble the head of an adult bird of the same species. Alternatively, the chick can be fed via a chute so that it is unable to see the person feeding it. The chick should preferably be reared with a sibling or, if this is not possible, with a chick of approximately the same age of another similar species but of the same genus (e.g., two members of the genus *Falco*).

(d) If the fledgling is to be used for falconry, it can then be fed directly by the human handler placing small pieces of meat directly into the mouth using blunt forceps. At this age the fledgling can be fed on chopped, surplus hatchery day-old chicks that have had the yolk sac removed or, alternatively, killed baby rats or freshly killed quail with the heads, wings, and guts removed. If any of these foods have been stored frozen, they must be fed fresh, immediately after defrosting. The meat should be dipped in normal saline and dusted with a suitable avian vitamin and mineral supplement. Very soon after this age the chick can be encouraged to feed from a saucer. Feed 3 to 4 times daily, and constantly check the crop for signs of impaction.

129 (a) This lesion looks like a fistula of the crop.

(b) It was confirmed as such by straightforward physical examination after the area had been cleaned with an antiseptic solution. In this case the lesion was due to external trauma, possibly by collision. Other cases in other species may be caused by internal perforation by an ingested sharp object (e.g., a spicule bone in a raptor) or faulty feed technique of fledglings.

(c) Treatment is by surgical repair. Both skin and the tissues of the crop should be sutured separately.

130 (a) Nothing can be done to restore the beak to a completely normal state. However, providing the tissues are kept clean and secondary infection is not allowed to become established, the beak will heal. Healing may be helped by suturing a strip of hydrophilic dressing (e.g., granuloflex) along the lesion. Sutures holding this should go through the premaxilla. Parental antibiotics should be used for a minimum of 2 to 3 weeks.

(b) The long-term prognosis is reasonable. Although the exact architecture of the beak on the affected side will not be reestablished, the duck will be able to feed.

131 (a) This orange-yellow, slightly nodular lesion is very suggestive of a xanthoma.

(b) This could be confirmed by fine-needle biopsy when vacuolated macrophages, cholesterol crystals, and multicellular giant cells would be expected to be seen.
(c) Medical treatment of this problem is not usually successful. Anion-exchange resins for hypercholesterolemia in humans are available, but these often have undesirable side effects and are not recommended for use in birds. For a lesion smaller than in the case illustrated, surgical removal using a monopolar wire electrode of a radiosurgical instrument is often successful. Nevertheless it is a wise precaution to apply a temporary tourniquet first, because these lesions can be quite vascular. Healing is by secondary intention, and a hydroactive dressing is best applied by suturing and bandaging during this period.
In the case illustrated amputation of the wing tip was necessary.

132 (a) This is a microfilarial larva of an adult nematode worm (Filarioidea). These larvae are an occasional finding in avian blood smears, and there is no pathologic effect linked to the occurrence of this stage of the parasite. One author has even seen these microfilaria in the anterior chamber of a parrot's eye. Filariasis can cause CNS problems in ostrich chicks (*Struthio camelus*).
(b) The adult forms are located in several body tissues, depending on the species of filaria (air sac, heart, subcutaneous tissue, blood vessels, etc.). Nevertheless, in most species pathogenicity appears to be low, because filaroid worms may be found in clinically healthy birds or incidentally at necropsy in falcons, passeriformes, and psittacine birds.

133 (a) These lesions are caused by *Knemidokoptes mutans,* a viviparous mite that lives permanently in the epidermis of the host. The infection is spread via direct contact transmission.
(b) Infections with *K. mutans* are seen in galliformes, especially in those birds kept in extensive husbandry systems. Infection is also occasionally diagnosed in zoologic specimens. Clinical signs can show in birds of 3 to 4 months of age, but distinct, visible scaly and crusted changes are only seen in older individuals as the disease slowly progresses. Because of the short life span in intensively kept poultry and measures such as regular disinfection and all-in-all-out management, the disease does not play a role in this type of husbandry.
(c) The crust should first be softened and removed with keratolytic agents. The legs should then be treated with an acarotoxic solution. Therapy should include asymptomatic birds, which may be carriers, as well as disinfection of the premises.

134 (a) This bird suffers from a spinal cord injury caused by a fracture or subluxation of the vertebral column or possibly a prolapse of an intervertebral disc. Diagnosis of spinal cord injuries in birds can be challenging, because myelograms are not practical in small birds and fractures of the vertebral column can be difficult to diagnose, especially in smaller species. Sometimes, callus formation several weeks after the injury is the only hint of such a fracture. An anatomic site of predilection for a fracture to occur is between the last free thoracic vertebra and synsacrum, which is the least stable site in the caudal part of the vertebral column. Prognosis is poor with fractures or injuries of the spinal cord; however, some birds do recover after several weeks.
(b) The bird is best placed in a quiet environment, preferably on soft material in a box to restrict movement, which will help to prevent further damage. Steroid or nonsteroidal anti-inflammatory injections can be useful in reducing edema and swelling at the site of the injury. If the bird is not able to pass feces because of cloacal paralysis, manual evacuation of the cloaca will be necessary. Provided that the bird shows no further disturbance of its general condition, it may be kept like this for some time. However, if no improvement is seen after several weeks, euthanasia will be necessary.

135 **(a)** This radiograph indicates a proximal fracture of the ulna, signs of healing (i.e., callus formation), and inhomogeneous structures with increased density in the medullary cavity and periosteal region of the bone. This is the radiographic appearance of an osteomyelitis, which is occasionally seen in combination with open or compound fractures or systemic infection. In the case of infected open wounds, ubiquitous bacteria, such as *Staphylococcus, E. coli* and *Pseudomonas* organisms can usually be found in osseous tissue. If osteomyelitis is caused by infection with mycobacteria, the development of multiple focal osteolytic and sclerotic lesions is a characteristic finding (see Fig. 156). A worrying complication of osteomyelitis in birds is infection of the respiratory system via the air sacs directly communicating with the pneumatic bone.

(b) Although therapy depends on an antibiotic sensitivity test, clindamycin is the antibiotic of choice for the best penetration of bony structures. Nevertheless, cephalosporins, enrofloxacin, tetracyclines, and chloramphenicol (best avoided if another antibiotic is suitable) can all be used in bone infection. Mycobacteria-induced osteomyelitis should not be treated (see answer to Fig. 156).

136 This illustration does not reveal any pathologic process. The two prominent white globular structures in the abdominal cavity are active, hypertrophic testes, a normal physiologic finding in male birds during the breeding season. Because of the distinct difference in the size of active and inactive testes, it is possible to gain information about the readiness and ability to mate by endoscopic examination of the genital tract. This is of interest if eggs are laid by the female but fail to hatch.

137 **A,** This radiograph reveals fractures in both tibiotarsal bones, which are the pathologic fractures of metabolic bone disease. In this case this was caused by an imbalance in the Ca:P ratio and insufficient vitamin D$_3$. This imbalance of the these three elements is common, especially in growing birds. The Ca:P ratio should be in the region of 1.5:1 to 2.5:1, and there is an overall increased need for an adequate calcium supply during growth.

The resorption of calcium in the small intestine depends on the presence of adequate vitamin D$_3$, without which calcium is poorly resorbed. In addition to this, an excessive supply of phosphorus leads to an increased renal elimination of calcium, which exacerbates the situation. Also hypovitaminosis A and a heavy intestinal parasite load may adversely affect the resorption of nutrients from the ingesta.

B, An unbalanced diet containing only seeds, cereals, and nuts. In such a diet the supply of some important vitamins (i.e., A and D$_3$) is poor, and the Ca:P ratio is low. Psittacine birds should be familiar with a much more varied diet that contains fruits and green vegetables, as well as seeds and cereals. *Cooked* pulses, minced carrot, celery, and pine nuts can all be fed. Peanuts, particularly when in the shell, are risky because they often contain fungal spores (particularly those of *Aspergillus* organisms). Oily seeds hold a lot of calories but are prone to turning rancid, which may be a contributory factor in hypovitaminosis E and resultant myopathy.

Once a psittacine bird is adapted to a certain diet, it can be very difficult to change its dietary habits. However, if changes are made slowly and carefully with patience and persistence, a more suitable diet can be introduced. Try feeding the bird at set times rather than *ad libitum*. Try mixing *small* quantities of the new item into the usual diet while gradually (over several weeks) weeding out the undesirable items. Parrots will often eat tidbits they see the owner or other birds eating. Sprouted pulses or seeds are often more acceptable.

138 Blood in the anterior chamber is termed *hyphema*. This results from damage to the iris, which usually occurs after a perforating corneal wound or some other type of head trauma. If this is the only pathologic eye alteration, as in the owl illustrated, it requires no treatment. The blood is usually absorbed within a few days.

139 (a) The increased bone density of the medullary cavity of both femurs and tibiotarsal bones indicates that this bird is in the egg-laying phase of its reproductive cycle. The caudal part of the abdomen is swollen, and the gizzard, proventriculus, and small intestine have all been displaced rostrally. Most of the abdominal air sacs have been obliterated. From these radiographic observations there would seem to be a space-occupying lesion in the caudal abdomen. The aspiration of 10 ml of fluid from this area indicates a possible ovarian cyst.
(b) This particular bird was given a single injection of 1.5 mg medroxyprogesterone to reduce ovarian activity. The bird was hospitalized for a week and the condition resolved.

140 (a) This bird looks as if it is grossly overweight. Although a normal blue-fronted Amazon weighs about 400 g, this bird's weight was more than double that figure. Because of excessive uncontrolled food consumption and quite inadequate exercise, obesity is commonly seen particularly in female caged birds. A predisposition to this condition is documented as occurring in rose-breasted cockatoos *(Cacatua leadbeateri* or *Eolophus roseicapillis)*, budgerigars and Amazon parrots. Diagnosis is made by palpation, inspection of the typical fat-induced swelling, and weighing the bird.
Lipomas are a common sequela to obesity, and this is probably the identity of the abnormal mass in the caudal abdomen. However, the mass could be a hernia, another kind of neoplasm, or a hematoma. Contrast radiography using barium contrast would be a wise precaution before surgery is contemplated. In extreme cases, such as the one illustrated, sudden death may occur as a result of fatty liver degeneration and liver rupture because of massive circulatory problems.
(b) Therapy consists of a general reduction of the calorific intake in the diet, particularly oil seeds. Low-fat foods, such as green vegetables and pulses, should be given and exercise increased (free flight, preferably in an aviary). The lipoma in the caudal area was surgically removed after 4 weeks when the bird's circulatory system seemed stable enough for anesthesia.

141 (a) These droppings look as if they are stained with blood.
(b) They could of course be colored from eating beet root, elderberries, or blackberries. A routine in-house test for the presence of blood can be performed. If the test is positive, the presence of blood may indicate a neoplasm (e.g., papilloma of the cloaca), tuberculosis, heavy metal poisoning (e.g., lead), bacterial enteritis, or impaction of the cloaca with a fecalith or possibly an egg. Direct visual or endoscopic examination will confirm or invalidate the latter diagnosis. Bacterial stains using both Gram's and acid-fast stains may help with the diagnosis. The diagnosis can also be supported by bacterial culture and a serum agglutination test for tuberculosis. Radiography may indicate lead poisoning, which can be confirmed by an assay of blood levels.
This bird was in fact a case of tuberculosis, which is consistent with the low body weight and normal appetite.

142 (a) The blackened structure is the partially necrotic tendon of the extensor digitorum lungus muscle.
(b) It is most important to first obtain a swab for bacteriologic culture, after which appropriate antibiotics can be used both locally and systemically. Secondly, the wound should be

thoroughly cleansed, preferably with a povidone-iodine solution. No attempt is made at this stage to suture any tissues. The most important procedure is to attempt to preserve the intact blood supply and encourage the development of an increased blood supply, particularly to the tendinous tissues that normally have little blood supply themselves. They are nourished from the surrounding tendon sheath. This objective is achieved by covering the sterilized area with a hydroactive dressing. This is changed every 3 to 4 days at first and then every 5 to 6 days. Active revascularization may take several weeks, and the tendon may adhere to the adjacent tendon sheath. When all tissue is well vascularized, repair of any ruptured tendon or tendon sheath can be performed with no. 4-0 polydioxanone as necessary. The tissues may heal without suturing, but it is a waste of time and counterproductive to try and suture tissues before there is a good blood supply.

During the whole healing period of probably several weeks the foot should be kept in a ball bandage so that the tendons are rested and there is less danger of them completely rupturing.

143 The tibiotarsal area of the leg appears bow shaped, and the intertarsal joint (the hock) appears abnormally flexed. From these observations it would appear that this fledgling has metabolic bone disease. (See the answer to Fig. 137.)

144 **(a)** This is a chronic herniation of the abdominal viscera, which has been left far too long by the owner without obtaining veterinary advice. The bird appears to be a female with the first signs of brown hypertrophy of the cere.

(b) Both this and the herniation are related to hormonal imbalance. Muscle weakness may be hormonally induced or may result from a faulty calcium metabolism. The aponeurosis of the abdominal muscles has split, and the descended abdominal viscera are supported by only the skin. This may have been precipitated by obstipation, cloacalithiasis, or egg-binding.

(c) Because the abdominal air sacs are in close association with the viscera this condition results in severe compromise of the respiratory system. The net result is that these birds are a bad anesthetic risk. Replacement of the organs will require great care and may require staging. The weakened abdominal wall should be supported using a surgical mesh. Oversuturing the repair with no. 4-0 nonchromic cat gut may help to encourage fibrosis. Chromic cat gut used in birds tends to cause too much inflammatory reaction and takes too long to be reabsorbed. The skin and muscle should be sutured with no. 3-0 polyglactin 910 swaged onto an atraumatic tapered-point needle. Strict asepsis and antibiotic cover for a minimum of 10 days is essential.

145 **(a)** There is ptosis of the bird's right upper eyelid, slight swelling of the right periorbital region, and a drooped right wing. In this case, ptosis is probably a consequence of trauma to the oculomotor nerve concurrent with the inflammatory swelling on the right side of the skull.

(b) The red color of the eyes is normal in older individuals of this species, because the eyes turn from yellow to red under the influence of sunlight with increasing age.

(c) Tonometry and a fluorescein-test should be performed to rule out ocular damage. Whole-body radiography, including the skull, would also be a wise precaution to indicate any skeletal damage. Regression of the swelling will usually result in normal function of the eyelid.

146 **(a)** The different forms of canary pox infection are as follows:
• Those exhibiting cutaneous crustlike lesions around the beak, on the legs and feet, and on any other featherless areas of the body. In chronic cases these lesions can progress to take on a tumorlike appearance.

• A mucosal form of the disease causes disruption to the mucosae of the beak, oropharynx, larynx, and trachea together with secondary infection.

• Although systemic pox infection leads to lesions mainly of the respiratory tract, hepatosis, splenomegaly, and inflammation of the small intestine may be found at necropsy.

(b) Respiratory signs, cutaneous or mucocutaneous lesions, or sudden death may be seen in different birds of an infected flock. Also, an infected bird may exhibit all the three forms of the disease simultaneously.

(c) A definitive diagnosis of pox virus is made through histopathologic examination of a biopsy sample to demonstrate the intracytoplasmic inclusions or Bollinger bodies in the epithelium of affected tissue. The virus can also be cultured from fecal samples.

(d) There is no risk of cross-species transmission of the virus to pigeons, because the virus tends to be species, or at most genera, specific. Very few avipox viral strains are known to cross the species barrier. Only other finches that hybridize with canaries are susceptible to canary pox infection.

147 This laterolateral radiograph shows a distinct overdistension of the abdominal air sacs. This feature is known as "air trapping." It often results from stenosis of the syringeal airway because of an obstructing mass producing a valvelike effect. The net result is an impediment to expiration and a build-up of pressure within the air sac system until the internal pressure is able to overcome the resistance caused by the obstruction. Air trapping is primarily seen with extensive mycosis of the respiratory tract.

148 In many cases such lesions are of iatrogenic origin. Bacterial infection following intramuscular injection is rarely seen in avian therapy. It is more frequently caused by the injection of irritating formulations (e.g., incompatible solvents) or tissue-damaging substances or repeated injections at the same injection site, resulting in muscle necrosis or necrotizing abscesses. Among those substances with a potential to cause muscular damage if administered intramuscularly (sometimes dependent on the formulation and species injected) are acyclovir, tylosin, erythromycin, various tetracyclines or doxycycline formulations, calcium EDTA, enrofloxacin, occasional sulfonamide preparations, and amphotericin B.

These lesions must be differentiated from the tumorlike changes caused by such viral infections as Marek's disease (probably does not occur in parrots), leukosis, and tuberculosis. In these latter cases, the lesions are often multiple and associated with additional clinical signs.

149 (a) The whole of the handler's right hand is grasping the bird's neck and throat, thereby risking compression of the respiratory tract and restricting breathing. The head, with the powerful beak, is not adequately restrained. Clutching the legs and feet in such a manner is unsatisfactory.

(b) The head can be controlled by encircling the proximal neck and submandibular area with the closed thumb and forefinger of the right hand or, better yet, placing gentle but firm pressure on the temporomandibular joints. The other fingers of the right hand exert no pressure but may help to control the carpometacarpal joint of the bird's right wing.

The legs should be held such that the index finger is placed between the patient's legs in the area of the distal tibiotarsus or tarsometatarsal region. The thumb and middle finger are then used to fixate the legs and if possible also the tips of the wings. Furthermore, the legs and neck should be carefully stretched and the bird held as close to the body as possible. This makes restraint safer and helps in minimizing defensive movement associated with the risk of leg fracture, especially in the smaller species.

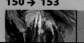
150 (a) The erythrocytes are characterized by marked hypochromasia of the cytoplasm, with some nuclei exhibiting polychromasia and others showing poikilocytosis and abnormal nuclear displacement.
In this bird, lead intoxication was suspected. Although hematologic changes do not necessarily occur, morphologic changes reported to be associated with this condition in the peripheral blood are numerous and include chromatin clumping, erythrocytic ballooning, basophilic stippling, cytoplasmic vacuolization, and increased mitosis. In birds, the findings typically include hemolytic aplastic anemia accompanied initially by a strong bone marrow response. In cases of severe liver disease, erythrocytes can mimic very closely the indications of lead poisoning. Distinctive but not pathognomonic erythrocyte changes develop within 2 to 3 days after lead ingestion.
(b) Radiography can be used to confirm the presence of lead in a bird. Alternatively, the estimation of the δ-aminolevulinic acid dehydrase (ALAD) activity, measured directly in the blood, has been shown to be a suitable and highly specific diagnostic test for lead intoxication.

151 There is an increase in soft tissue density in the abdomen and the ventriculus has been displaced cranially. Furthermore, an increase in the density of the long bones together with inhomogeneous areas in the endosteal regions of the bones can be seen. This increased density is termed *medullary bone* and is a normal physiologic occurrence during the egg-laying period of the reproductive cycle. The increased medullary bone provides a reserve of calcium necessary for the production of the egg shell and is under the influence of androgens, estrogens, and parathyroid hormone.
However, the abnormal formation of medullary bone occurs in combination with various cysts, egg-binding, or neoplasms of the ovary or, rarely, the testes.
In this bird the increased abdominal soft tissue density together with the distension of the abdomen was subsequently diagnosed as a laminated egg after ultrasonography.

152 (a) A small number of coccidial oocysts is usually of little significance. However, counts above 3000 oocysts/g of feces can indicate a moderate infection, and counts over 20,000 oocysts/g demonstrate a severe infection. *Capillaria* spp., or hairworms, are far more pathogenic, burrowing into the wall of the alimentary tract and causing severe diarrhea and occasional vomiting. Infection with a relatively small number of capillarial worms can result in death in pigeons. Infection with these worms is common.
Parasitologic findings may only underlie the major cause of a disease problem, which could be bacterial (e.g., salmonellosis or chlamydial infection), or viral (e.g., pigeon herpesvirus; infectious esophagitis; intranuclear inclusion body hepatitis; pigeon adenovirus infection, which is often asymptomatic; or paramyxovirus infection).
Candidiasis may also occur as a secondary infection, and the clinician should not overlook such parasites as *Hexamita, Trichomonas, or Toxoplasma*.
(b) The parasitologic burden in the bowel may have contributed to the disease process by interfering with the absorption of vitamins, proteins, and other nutrients. Apart from further laboratory investigation, postmortem examination, and so on to identify the root cause of the problem, antiparasitic therapy must be instituted and the diet supplemented with vitamins and minerals to improve the overall health of the birds.

153 (a) Both elbow joints show signs of congenital subluxation. There are also signs of erosion of the bone and some exostosis, all of which would militate against the resolution of normal joint action.

(b) Successful surgical treatment of a luxated elbow joint in birds is difficult and depends on rigid stabilization, under general anesthetic, of the correctly repositioned radius, ulna, and humerus. This is achieved using Kirschner-type wires and an external fixator. To have any chance of success this should be carried out within 72 hours of the original trauma. The device should be kept in position for at least 7 to 15 days. Limited but voluntary cage exercise is then allowed, which may be assisted if practical with passive movement of the joint for another 5 to 14 weeks to encourage an increase in the range of movement. After this the bird can be placed in a free-flight cage. Prognosis is always doubtful.

154 (a) These worms are most likely to be of the *Ascaridia* spp.
(b) The life cycle is direct; therefore the bird has most likely become infected through a contaminated food or water supply. Some psittacine species, such as budgerigars *(Melopsittacus undulatus)*, are also coprophagic. Ascarid eggs are particularly resistant to disinfection and survive well in moist environments, so clean, dry surroundings reduce the chances of infection.
(c) Before death this bird exhibited weight loss, although appetite was maintained and in fact seemed to have increased. The droppings were very fluid, with little fecal content. Death was due to bowel impaction.
(d) If such cases of massive worm infestation are diagnosed antemortem, care should be taken to administer liquid paraffin (mineral oil) or olive oil (by gavage tube) simultaneously with the anthelmintic (fenbendazole or levamisole), otherwise impaction can still occur after the death of a large number of nematode worms.

155 (a) This is a honey buzzard *(Pernis apivorus)*. It may occasionally be mistaken for a common buzzard *(Buteo buteo)*, but the honey buzzard has a slimmer head and narrow, longish nares (nares in common buzzards are much more triangular). The feet and toes are also more slender.
(b) The honey buzzard uses its feet and toes to dig and tear out the larvae, pupae, and imagines of wasps and bumblebees. Other insects, such as beetles and locusts, as well as small mammals, reptiles, amphibians, and young birds are also taken, particularly if there is a shortage of staple food.
(c) Some institutions, such as bird rehabilitation centres, which are more frequently confronted with the problem of feeding these birds, keep a stock of frozen honeycombs. If these are not available, dead mice or surplus hatchery chicks can be offered. Some honey buzzards readily accept these, but others will not. In the latter case, plants blighted with insects, boiled eggs, and ripe fruit such as apples, bananas, or even peas may be accepted.

156 (a) Normal appetite in combination with weight loss tends to indicate a consumptive disease. Birds are quite likely to suffer from tuberculosis or neoplasms. The radiograph shows an osteomyelitis that presents as areas of increased translucence that can be seen in several of the long bones.
(b) To confirm a diagnosis of tuberculosis, serologic testing using *Mycobacterium avium* antigen is of little value (false-negative results and cross-reactions are possible). Many birds infected with mycobacteriosis exhibit an increased white cell count. A biopsy of the affected tissue together with histopathology and bacterial culture is the only reliable method.
This particular kestrel did in fact have tuberculosis, which is often associated with arthritis, osteomyelitis, and tubercle formation in the muscles of falconiformes and accipitriformes. In most species of birds, granuloma formation is usually localized to the intestines and the reticuloendothelial organs, but any organ may be affected.

(c) There is no safe and effective therapy for birds with *Mycobacterium avium* infections. Because of the zoonotic potential of *Mycobacterium avium* and the lack of an appropriate treatment for infected humans, euthanasia should be considered for infected birds.

157 **(a)** **A,** Subcutaneous injection of fluid into the lateral flank. The operator should be careful not to perforate both layers of skin, because they lie very close together with little intervening tissue. **B,** Interosseous injection of fluid into the medullary cavity of the ulna. In this method, a suitable cannula with a stylet is placed in the bone cavity by inserting the needle through the distal end of the bone and gently pushing it with a slight rotational movement proximally. If fluid can be injected easily without causing a subcutaneous swelling, the cannula is then taped in place and the injection continued.

(b) Subcutaneous injection has the advantage of providing a comparatively large amount of fluid as a depot for subsequent relatively slow absorption. This method of administration should consequently be primarily used in cases of mild dehydration or for maintenance fluid therapy. It is recommended that the total amount of fluid is distributed over several sites (e.g., up to 10 ml/kg body weight per site with a total maximum of 20 ml/kg). If large quantities of fluid are required immediately (e.g., in cases of shock or severe dehydration) or fluid must be given over a longer period, the use of an interosseous cannula can be an alternative to intravenous injection. High rates of resorption can be achieved and, compared with intravenous application, maintaining a continuous fluid administration over a longer period (i.e., 2 to 3 days) is less difficult when using an interosseous injection.

158 **(a)** The avian fundus varies in color among different species.

(b) In birds the retina is avascular and the optic nerve is very short. In diurnal birds the cones outnumber the rods. The density of cones is greater (approximately $\times$ 2) than in the human retina. Rods that are reactive to the intensity of light are far more numerous in nocturnal birds, and several rods are connected to one ganglion cell, making the eye even more sensitive to light of low intensity. In contrast, in the eye of diurnal birds, one cone synapses with a single ganglion cell, so that each cone has a direct connection to the visual cortex and consequently visual acuity is greater. Covering the area of the optic nerve is a pleated vane-like vascular melanotic projection termed the *pecten,* which can be seen running diagonally across the centre of the illustration. There is considerable interspecies variation in its size and structure, but it always protrudes into the fairly fluid vitreous humor and is believed to be associated with the provision of oxygen and nutrients to the avascular retina. There is no tapetum lucidum, but most birds have well-developed fovea and some have two foveate areas in which the cones are more densely concentrated.

(c) There are many different causes for retinal pathology, and many adverse changes can be recognized. For example, destruction of rods and cones can result from the development of focal scar tissue. A retinitis resulting in either transudate or exudate can be serious. It can be persistent and at the very least irreversible. Also, a retinitis may occur as a result of any inflammatory process in other parts of the eye and lead eventually to detachment of the retina. A retinitis resulting from toxoplasmosis has been documented in canaries *(Serinus canaria).* A chorioretinitis may be the result of a nutritional deficiency such as hypovitaminosis A. Retinal bleeding from damaged choroidal vessels or the fragile pecten is commonly seen and can result from trauma. A reovirus infection has also been implicated in psittacine birds.

159 **(a)** There is a healing fracture of the right ulna with a well-developed bony callus that indicates the injury could have occurred at least 3 weeks previously. The obvious midshaft fracture of the left tibiotarsus is not healing so well. Although there is plenty of bony cal-

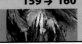

lus on the medial aspect, this is irregular in density. The endosteal bone at the fracture site, besides being irregular, lacks overall density. Also, the distal segment shows an area of sclerosis. This indicates probable infection and an osteomyelitis. The soft tissues of the leg are also swollen.

(b) Swabs for microbiologic culture and antibiotic sensitivity should be obtained from this lesion before surgery. The wound should be enlarged and curetted, and the bone should be flushed daily to remove necrotic debris and provide good drainage. It would be inadvisable to close the wound until the tissue is healthy and free from infection. During this period the fracture site is best supported in an external splint. Any attempt at using an implanted fixator could result in further infection of the bone.

A lateral radiograph may help to locate the air gun pellet more accurately. However, unless the pellet is found to be near the surface it may be wiser to leave it in situ because lead poisoning is unlikely to result unless the lead is within the gastrointestinal tract.

160 (a) The plasma color and clarity provide a useful index of the degree of hemolysis that is most likely to result from a poor sampling technique or from prolonged sample storage.

(b) True hemoglobinemia is rarely encountered in birds. When seen, this condition is most often associated with heavy metal poisoning (i.e., plumbism, zinc, and cadmium). Apart from an artefactual hemolysis secondary to improper handling of blood samples, the condition also occurs in various physiologic conditions or disease processes.

In birds, normal plasma color varies from clear to a yellowish tinge, but this is influenced by overall nutrition and particularly by vitamin supplementation. Carotinoids and other feather pigments are normal plasma constituents in some avian species. A white, cloudy, or milky appearance to the plasma may indicate lipemia (commonly seen in postprandial and obese birds, laying birds, hepatopathies, and hypothyroidism). Egg yolk peritonitis may turn the plasma a thick creamy, orange and mimic lipemia. Yellow plasma, commonly seen in yellow and green budgerigars (*Melopsittacus undulatus*) and in brightly colored birds in general, should not be mistakenly considered an indication of jaundice. Despite the high incidence of liver disease, clinical icterus is rarely seen in birds, but its occurrence is more likely to be seen in macaws (*Ara* spp.).

Total plasma protein values in conjunction with erythrocyte indices are a useful diagnostic aid for the assessment of a patient's general state of nutrition, hydration, or anemia but are of little value when looked at in isolation, because there is considerable variation in healthy birds. Although the determination of plasma protein levels will help to evaluate the severity and progression of the disease process, changes in the various components of plasma protein merely suggest that trends are by no means pathognomonic. Because fibrinogen is an acute phase protein, its level is one of the most useful tests for confirming infection and other inflammatory diseases and also for following the patient's progress and response to therapy.

Besides an examination of the stained blood film, the measurement of the packed cell volume/hematocrit is considered to be most important in avian hematology. In adult birds, a reduction below 35% of normal indicates anemia. Values greater than 60% are found in dehydration or polycythemia secondary to erythropoiesis, respiratory, renal disease, or cardiac disease.

The height of the buffy coat gives a rough but quick estimation of the total leukocyte count. However, in avian blood, half of the buffy coat is composed of thrombocytes. Normal birds have buffy coats less than 1%; high white cell counts may be reflected by buffy coats of over 1% to 2%. Motile blood parasites (microfilaria, trypanosomes) may be detected in the plasma above the buffy coat.

161 (a) These cells are maturing erythrocytes. Each cell passes through a *continuously develop-ing* process. For the sake of convenience, individual cells are classified into named stages of development. As a result of this *artificial static* scheme, the terminology and even the defi-nitions given for different categories of erythrocytic development vary in the literature. Classification of maturing cells is commonly based on cell shape (which usually corre-sponds to that of the cell nucleus), cell size, nucleocytoplasmic ratio, staining reaction (dependent on a particular nomenclature), and microtexture of both nucleus and cyto-plasm. As a rule, early developing cells are larger, predominantly round with a clearly visi-ble nucleus, and characterized by a high nucleus:cytoplasm ratio. Mature cells and those in the later stages of maturation have more condensed, deeply basophilic nuclear chromatin. During maturation the cytoplasm has a contrary tendency to become more eosinophilic.
(b) All stages of developing erythroid cells, which includes the proerythroblast, basophilic erythroblast, polychromatic erythroblast, and orthochromatic erythroblast may occasion-ally be found in the peripheral circulation.
(c) Morphologic differentiation does not cause any difficulties beyond the proerythroblast. Reliable classification of stages next to mature cells may require staining methods other than Giemsa staining. When the immature erythrocyte is stained by vital dyes, such as new methylene blue or brilliant cresol blue, the cell develops a bluish stippling or reticular pat-tern. This reticulum results from the staining of ribosomal RNA, which is abundant in immature cells. Both the concentration of the stain and the staining time affect the amount of the reticulum observed. The maturation stage most often identified as reticulocyte in conventionally stained preparations is the polychromatophilic erythroblast, but basophilic and orthochromatic erythroblasts and the mature erythrocytes may also contain a reticu-lum. Another index for estimating the incidence of immature erythrocytes is the polychro-matophilic index. This is the percentage of the number of *distinctly* polychromatic cells pre-sent in Romanowsky-stained peripheral blood smears. This can provide a qualitative, com-parative measurement of the erythropoietic response.
(d) The significance of the finding in the case illustrated is that it is a normal physiologic finding. The number of immature cells, those penultimate to mature erythrocytes (i.e., orthochromatic erythroblasts or reticulocytes) predominating by far, usually do not exceed 5% to 10% of the total red blood cells. Immature red cells are more common in young birds and in species of small body size. Reticulocyte counts greater than 50% are not uncommon in severe, nonregenerative anemias. As can be shown in experimental phenylhydrazine intoxication, even advanced maturation of erythrocyte cells does not preclude (peripheral) cell division.

162 (a) Both these chicks are sitting down on their hocks. In the bird on the left the digits appear to be rotated medially. Although both birds appeared to be feathered normally, there is a distinct lack of any pigmentation in both of them.
(b) The birds appear to be suffering from a marginal but multiple vitamin and mineral deficiency.

163 This bird has swallowed at least three, if not four, fishhooks, which have become lodged in the proventriculus and gizzard. Although it would not be impossible to remove these hooks, it would be difficult and time-consuming. This is a wild bird, and it is ethically debatable whether it is right for a bird such as this to be subjected to a major surgical pro-cedure and then be hospitalized during the convalescent period. These birds are a common species that is not in danger of becoming extinct. The birds normally feed on a mainly veg-etable diet of seeds, fruits, grass, leaves, and moss, with a little animal matter, such as insects, earthworms, slugs, snails, and occasionally fish. The fact that this particular bird has swallowed three or four fishhooks indicates it has a particular liking for fish or at least pond-bottom vegetation with entangled fish hooks. Even if the bird was finally released away from its original habitat it is quite capable of returning, because some individuals of this species do migrate. It could then again become affected by the same problem. Euthanasia is the wise decision in this case.

164 (a) Because of the gross nature of this lesion it would be obvious that the prolapse is not due to the following causes:
• Simple prolapse of the cloacal mucus membrane (i.e., cloacitis resulting from an infection or allergic reaction
• Virally induced papillomata (seen particularly in some psittacine species, such as Amazons and macaws)
• Any other type of neoplasm, such as adenoma
• Fecal urate impaction of the cloaca
If there is a history of recent egg laying, the prolapse could have resulted in a prolapse of the oviduct with a retained egg. However, in the case illustrated the shape of the prolapse does not look as if it contains an egg (radiography would help in the diagnosis). The history of chronic gram-negative enteritis indicated by loose droppings and green staining and/or pastiness around the vent may indicate a prolapse of the rectum, possibly containing an intussusception of the intestine. In a case such as that illustrated the bird may be found on the floor of its cage showing obvious tenesmus or even paresis of the legs.
(b) A bird in such a condition will be in a severe state of shock and will require immediate fluid therapy, warmth, and possibly intravenous corticosteroids. The prolapsed viscus must be kept moist with warm saline (390 C [102° F]). If an egg can be detected within the prolapse, this can be first extracted by incision of the oviductal wall. After the incision is sutured and corticosteroid cream applied (to reduce the inflammatory reaction and act as a lubricant), it may be possible to replace the prolapsed oviduct using a blunt probe, such as the end of a clinical thermometer. Failing this, amputation of a prolapsed oviduct is the only solution.
(c) The case illustrated is an intussusception. The only way to surgically resolve these cases is via a coleotomy and then *very gentle* traction on the intestine to withdraw this and the prolapse back into the abdomen. This can then be retained in position with either a rib or a sternal cloacopexy.

165 (a) Because the matted feathering involves the feathers on the crown of the head and not just around the eyes, this is most likely to have been caused by excessive production of oropharyngeal mucus.
Had the matting of the feathers been confined to just the areas surrounding the eyes this would most likely have been due to epiphora. The matted feathering on the top of the head is caused by the bird flicking its head in an attempt to rid itself of excessive mucus in the mouth, so that the string of mucus ends up on the head.
Excessive production of oral mucus in the budgerigar is mostly due to an infection with *Trichomonas* or *Candida* organisms, but in other species of birds *Capillaria* infection should also be considered. Sometimes these infections are superimposed on an underlying *Chlamydia* infection.
(b) Confirmation of the diagnosis is by the examination of a freshly obtained and wet-mounted crop wash for motile trichomoniasis. For identification of *Candida* organisms the sample should be dried, fixed, and stained with methylene blue or a Romanowsky stain (preferably one of the modified quick Wright's stains) that will also stain fixed trichomonads.

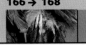

166 (a) This was an exophthalmus resulting from retrobulbar hemorrhage.
(b) An exophthalmus may be the result not only of trauma (e.g., a bite in pet birds, as in the case illustrated) but also of an infectious process or a retrobulbar neoplasm. An abnormally positioned globe caused by a retrobulbar hematoma is not uncommon in wild birds as a result of a collision trauma.
(c) Such hematomata are often absorbed without treatment. However, if this condition should become secondarily infected with bacteria or if a unilateral exophthalmus is caused by a primary bacterial infection, the prognosis is guarded and the success of antibiotic treatment is uncertain.

167 (a) This is the residuum of a *Microfilarium*. Microfilaria are frequently diagnosed in (imported) exotic birds. Although normally detected in the circulating blood, they may also be found in organ impression smears, even if these have not been adequately stained.
(b) Affected birds may show lameness or loss of feathers (induced by subcutaneous edema and mostly noninflammatory nodule formation) together with a reddish-blue discoloration of the skin.
Cardiovascular lesions include thickening of the pulmonary arteries, pulmonary arterial thrombosis, pericardial effusions, and myocardial degeneration. In these cases the end result is often fatal. The premonitory signs comprise a reluctance to fly, anorexia, and emaciation. In falcons (Falconides) the adult worms are documented as having precipitated an air sacculitis. Microfilaria have been incriminated in the induction of anemia and hemosiderosis. Larvae may concentrate in great numbers in the capillaries, resulting in seizures (and other CNS signs in ostrich chicks) and death.
Amicrofilaraemic infection (occult filariasis) is thought to be accidental. In these cases, vascular changes have been attributed, but not proven, to be caused by *Microfilaria* organisms. Ocular manifestation of a single adult worm has been shown to cause iridocyclitis, synechia, and mydriasis.
Because the disease potential of the hematozoa does not necessarily correlate with parasitemia, blood smear examination should be combined with capillary tube centrifugation where indicated (see the answer to Fig. 160). Besides being more sensitive for the detection of hematozoa, the technique yields viable parasites, and, in the case of microfilaria, the larval sheath, which is an important characteristic for genus identification, can more easily be detected.
(c) The pathogenicity of avian filaroids is commonly considered to be low (except in ostrich chicks). Clinical manifestation has been documented for members of the orders Psittaciformes, Anseriformes, Passeriformes; the infraorder Falconides; and ostriches (Struthioniformes). Specific clinical signs are mostly tissue-oriented. Adult worms (*Serratospiculum* spp.) have been reported to involve the cutis, subcutis, and muscular skeletal system (especially the hock joints, metatarsal region, and digits).

168 There is a general overall increase in soft tissue density of the whole abdominal area and of the right lung. The abdominal and posterior thoracic air sacs are almost totally obliterated, although the clavicular air sac and certainly its two extrathoracic diverticula look quite clear. The ventriculus with its contained grit has been slightly displaced to the left and slightly rostrally. From this it can be deduced that there is a space-occupying lesion of the abdominal or, more strictly, coelomic cavity. Because there is no increase in medullary bone, this bird is not in the egg-laying phase of its reproductive cycle, so the assumption is that this bird has either a massive neoplasm (which is possible because often cachexia together with a tumor will result in a body weight within the normal range, 230 to 540 g) or an abdominal abscess.

Euthanasia was performed, and at autopsy a large abscess measuring approximately 4 × 2 cm and filled partly with inspissated pus and partly with liquid pus was found occupying most of the coelom and involving the right lung. *E. coli* was cultured.

169 **(a)** On the left is a heterophil, on the right is an eosinophil.

(b) As a rule, heterophils are the most common granulocytes seen in all avian species. Heterophils have a colorless cytoplasm (unless toxic changes or staining artifacts have occurred), whereas that of eosinophils is a clear pale blue. This is not obvious in this particular illustration. In heterophils the cytoplasmic granules are fusiform or rod shaped, but they may be spherical in some avian species (and vice versa in the eosinophilic granulocytes).

(c) Because heterophilic cytoplasmic granules will disintegrate in aqueous solutions, their shape is influenced by the tonicity of the staining solution. Breakdown of the cytoplasmic rods will give an orange or pink color to the cytoplasm. On the other hand, in the eosinophils, the granules are unaffected by aqueous solutions and tend to be more evenly distributed throughout the cytoplasm compared with those in heterophils. In heterophils the nucleus is often partially hidden by the cytoplasmic granules. In eosinophils, the nucleus appears blue, shows dense chromatin clumps and is usually bilobed, the number of lobes being normally less than that of the heterophil.

Overall, there is considerable interspecific variation resulting in numerous deviations from the basic morphology of avian eosinophils and heterophils even in bird taxa that are closely related phylogenetically. A thorough scanning of the slide before initiating a cell count will usually permit a distinction to be made. Because the eosinophilic staining affinity of the cytoplasmic granules does not differ greatly from that of the heterophil granules, differentiation from heterophil granulocytes, especially in the abnormal hemogram, may prove to be difficult and should be more reliably based on cell morphology rather than on staining affinity.

(d) Regarding degranulation, the durability of the granulocytes is directly proportional to the size and/or state of health of the bird.

(e) In many cases, the granulocytes of small, heavily diseased birds rupture easily and affect the accuracy of a white blood cell count. All granulocytes have a tendency to lose their cytoplasmic granules in blood films made from stored samples or during inadequate fixation. Degranulation resulting from heterophil or eosinophil activation (i.e., in toxic cells) is often seen in severe systemic infection. The toxic cellular process proceeds through dark blue granulation, reduction in cell size together with cytoplasmic basophilia, and vacuolization followed by nuclear hypersegmentation, then karyorrhexis and karyolysis. Finally the architecture of the cell is completely disrupted.

170 **(a)** This radiograph shows signs of a dilated proventriculus with retained ingesta, possibly including some grit. These radiographic signs together with the clinical history indicate a diagnosis of psittacine neuropathic gastric proventricular dilation (also called *macaw wasting disease* and *psittacine myenteric ganglioneuritis*).

(b) This condition has been documented in many species of parrots other than macaws. It may also occur in other taxa and is now confirmed by British and American workers to be caused by a virus that destroys the autonomic ganglia of the myenteric plexus, heart, and CNS. However, it should be stressed that as yet there is no diagnostic test that can 100% confirm a diagnosis in the live bird. Common differential diagnoses with the same radiographic and clinical signs may indicate an infection with yeast organisms or possibly tapeworms.

171 **(a)** The differential diagnoses of cloacal prolapse are presented in the answer to Fig. 164.

(b) Accurate diagnosis will certainly require a thorough visual inspection performed under a general anesthetic. Endoscopy not only of the cloaca but also the oropharynx and esophagus may be necessary. Many papillomavirus-induced neoplasms of psittacine birds also affect the whole gastrointestinal tract, including the bile duct. Contrast radiography may also help in the final diagnosis. Application to the lesion of 5% acetic acid (which will turn white in the case of a papilloma) may also help differential diagnosis. Although virally induced cloacal papillomas occur in many species of psittacine birds, they are particularly common in Amazon parrots. If lesions are found in both upper and lower alimentary tracts, this will almost certainly be a papilloma caused by virus infection. However, a definitive diagnosis can only be reached after using histopathology. This particular case proved to be a benign adenoma.

172 Culture of a fecal sample may reveal organisms that are not the primary etiologic agent of the disease. Often the bacteria cultured are secondary invaders. Potential pathogens in psittacine birds are gram-negative bacteria, such as *Klebsiella* spp., *Pseudomonas* spp., and *Escherichia coli*. If these are found in large numbers in the fecal sample and in almost pure culture together with the relevant clinical signs, then they are probably the primary pathogen. On the other hand, routine fecal cultures may fail to diagnose pathogens such as *Mycobacteria* spp. or *Salmonella* spp. More specific cultural methods are necessary to demonstrate these organisms. It is always wise to supplement bacterial culture with a smear stained with Gram's stain and also one stained with Ziehl-Neelsen for acid-fast organisms.

173 **(a)** This bird shows a subluxation of the left humeral head.
(b) Careful comparison of left and right sides prompts suspicion of atrophy of the pectoral muscles on the affected side. This would indicate that the duration of the injury has been several days.
(c) These cases are not necessarily hopeless, but they do require urgent surgical attention.
(d) The tendon of the supracoracoideus muscle is usually detached from the dorsal surface of the proximal humerus subsequent to an avulsion fracture of the lesser tuberosity. This should be sutured back into position using no. 2-0 polypropylene nylon, polydioxanone, wire or, in a larger bird, lag screws. The wing must be immobilized with a figure-8 bandage for at least 2 weeks after surgery.

174 **(a)** This is a common nighthawk *(Chordeiles minor)* belonging to the family Caprimulgidae (i.e., the nightjars).
(b) The bird's normal breeding range extends over the whole of North America from the southern Yukon in northern Canada and southern Alaska in the United States to southern of Mexico.
(c) During autumn these birds migrate to Argentina. The conjecture is that during migration the bird became caught in a fast-moving westerly North Atlantic weather pattern and was blown off course, a common occurrence for many North American migrant species.
(d) After a thorough clinical examination, including radiography, a parasitologic screen, and a check of the plumage, the bird was maintained on a diet principally of wax moth larvae *(Galleria mellonella)*. The bird's normal diet consists of moths, beetles, and crickets caught in flight.

175 **(a)** The precise identity of the cell in the group of three could not be determined. It is considered to be a basophilic granulocyte, because no (normally appearing) basophil granulocytes could be detected and other cell types in this smear did not show any abnormal morphology. Along with pathologic changes, artifacts resulting from improper processing of

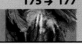

the sample should be taken into account. As mentioned in the answer to Fig. 169, a thorough initial scanning of the slide before final evaluation will usually help to judge the scale of any alterations caused by faulty processing and will help in avoiding a false diagnosis. The normal mature basophil is slightly smaller than the heterophil. The cytoplasm is colorless, and the variably numbered granules are strongly basophilic (i.e., blue-violet to black). Basophils tend to be spherical cells with a round, nonlobed, occasionally indented, and centrally or laterally located nucleus.

The nucleus is usually masked by the basophilic granules. These may appear to bulge at the periphery, giving the cell a blackberry-like appearance. The nuclear chromatin is not heavily condensed. The penetration of Wright's stain, found to be poor in the heterophil nucleus, is practically nil in the basophils.

(b) Regarding pathologic significance, abnormal basophilic granules may occur with the use of EDTA, Wright's stain, or other alcohol-solubilizers, aqueous stains, or fixatives. Consequently, morphologic changes in these cells have not proven helpful in the assessment of the avian patient's clinical state.

(c) Although more common in avian than in mammalian blood, basophils are still rare in the peripheral circulation of most clinically normal birds, with the possible exception of certain *Amazona* spp., finches, and all small birds. Basophilia may be associated with respiratory disease and tissue necrosis, particularly if they are of a long-term or chronic nature.

(d) The group of four cells are thrombocytes. Morphologic transformations associated with clotting or a mostly chronic state of disease are indicated by rounding up of both the thrombocyte cell and nucleus, cytoplasmic vacuolization, breakdown of the granules, and *aggregation of the cells*. The cytoplasm changes color from pale blue to reddish-violet or orange. These changes often aid in the identification of thrombocytes. By observing the cellular aggregates one may be able to appraise the quality of the sample, which may influence the estimates and counts of all representative cells.

176 (a) All the parrots (psittaciformes) have zygodactyl feet, that is, they have two forward-directed toes (digits II and III) and two backward-directed toes (digits I and IV). This type of foot has evolved as an aid to climbing and, particularly in some parrots, as a grasping foot to hold food.

The extensor tendons run along the dorsal surfaces of the phalanges, and the flexor tendons are on the ventral surface. Collateral ligaments hold the individual phalanges in position. There are also small intrinsic muscles that supplement the main extensor and flexor muscles. In the case illustrated all four digits (including I and IV) are directed forward on the left side (i.e., the bird's right foot). On the bird's left foot, digit IV is directed medially, interfering with the normal flexion of digit I.

(b) Subluxation of these maldirected digits has occurred between their articulation with the tarsometatarsus and phalanx number one of all the affected digits. The lateral ligaments have either ruptured or been abnormally slack. If the problem had been noticed when the bird was young and some attempt made to splint these joints, it may have been possible to correct the situation. However, not only have the joint surfaces become eroded but the tension on the tendons have become adjusted by shortening of the muscle fibers so that permanent resolution of this problem is almost impossible.

177 (a) There is an obvious healing fracture of the right coracoid. There is some involvement of the scapula, but the humerus appears to be all right except for some slight longitudinal rotation. This may be due to contraction of the pectoralis muscle, which shows some evidence of reduction in size (i.e., atrophy). This is probably disuse atrophy.

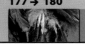

(b) Providing there is no interference with the tendon of the supracoracoideus muscle as it passes through the foramen trioseum this bird may be able to fly again. Gulls are primarily gliders, so as long as the bird can get airborne with the aid of a slight breeze and as long as there is no loss of extension of the wing (resulting in loss of lift) on the affected side, this bird will manage. This type of injury is much more serious in species that are strong, active flyers, such as pigeons, ducks, and falcons.
(c) Black-headed gulls are normally found well inland all over continental Europe, except Spain and Italy, even as far as Vienna.

178 (a) It is impossible by only a simple visual examination to make an exact diagnosis and hence give an accurate prognosis on any lesion, be it superficial or otherwise. This lesion did in fact turn out to be a capillary hemangioma. Although unlike hemangiosarcomas (from which they may be difficult to differentiate cytologically), these tumors do not metastasize. They do however bleed profusely if traumatized and during surgery.
(b) This lesion should be surgically removed (or lanced and curetted if during surgery it appears to be an abscess), and the harvested specimens should be sent for histopathology, no matter how small the lesion looks.

179 This is a case of chronic uveitis. After an injury to the iris, an anterior synechia (i.e., attachment of the iris to the cornea) or a posterior synechia (attachment of the iris to the lens) is likely to occur. Infectious disease that may be either primary or secondary may spread from the iris to the ciliary body and the choroidea, resulting in an irido-cyclito-chorioditis, otherwise known as a *generalized uveitis*. Besides blood, cell detritus and protein may accumulate in the anterior chamber, giving the pupil and iris a "dirty, foggy" appearance.
Open, dilated pupils may only be temporary and the result of minor trauma to the visual pathways or the cortex (e.g., after retinal or optic nerve damage). Alternatively, mydriasis with a fixed unresponsive pupil is also seen after infections and traumatic insults that may cause an anterior synechia. Another possible cause of mydriasis are local or systemic intoxications (e.g., disinfectants, lead poisoning, etc.). Although acute disease processes are often accompanied by epiphora, hemorrhage, exudate, and oversensitivity to light (causing miosis), chronic forms of an anterior uveitis may be associated with clinical signs such as a wide unresponsive pupil and synechia, as in the bird illustrated.

180 (a) This falcon shows bilateral polydactylism. There are two additional digits originating from the tarsometatarsal region of each leg. This bird was unable to walk properly. There would have been no chance of survival in its natural habitat, and euthanasia was performed.
(b) Congenital defects can occur during the incubation period as a result of many factors, among which are alimentary deficiency of the hen bird; physical, infectious, or chemical injury to the developing embryo; mutations; and disturbances of cell division. Hereditary defects in captive avian species may in some cases be related to intensive inbreeding to achieve special color or physical mutations not found in wild birds (e.g., the wild budgerigar is mostly green and yellow, but domestic specimens come in a variety of colors; the same applies to cockatiels, love birds, and the various types of canaries and fancy pigeons). Such manipulation by breeders can lead to or increase the incidence of various pathologic manifestations, such as feather abnormalities (feather cysts, "feather dusters"), skeletal disorders, ocular anomalies, and possibly an increased incidence of neoplasms in budgerigars (age may also be a factor). In wild birds, any hereditary disorders that have an adverse influence on their finding of food, food intake, mobility, or fertility are eliminated by the death

or failure to breed of the affected bird and consequently are not passed on to their offspring as is sometimes the case in companion birds. However, some mutations that do not affect survival in a wild habitat, such as total or partial leucism, are recorded.

181 Drugs can be administered in medicated food or in drinking water to birds kept in large flocks or to several birds in a group. This method is useful when numbers of birds must be caught for individual dosing, catching of individuals may result in unacceptable levels of stress, or catching an individual may be difficult (e.g., ratites, particularly cassowaries [*Casuariidae* spp.] which can be very dangerous). However, when medicating both food or water, the palatability of the prepared mixture and consequent reduction in food or water intake may be critical in very sick birds. Also, if the water containing the drug is in an environment with a high temperature and low humidity, considerable evaporative loss could occur, resulting in an increased concentration of the drug. Another factor to consider is that some species of birds are partially xerophilic and can survive without water for several days, whereas other species cannot go without water for very long (e.g., compare budgerigars and canaries). Birds in a flock are also themselves individuals, and, although some will eat or drink, others will not.
Single birds can be dosed orally via gavage. The type (metal, plastic, rubber) and the length of gavage tube will depend on the species. Some single species of birds can also be given tablets or capsules. All of these methods for single birds make medication much more precise. The correct dose is administered at set times to achieve a much more consistent level of the drug in the bird's body. However, resorption from the intestines must be taken into account if systemic disease is to be treated (e.g., aminoglycosides and amphotericin-B are not absorbed from the gastrointestinal tract; absorption of ampicillin is poor and erratic). Sometimes these limitations can be overcome by using subcutaneous, intramuscular, or intravenous routes.

182 **(a)** This disorder is known as "splay leg" and is seen in nestlings and fledglings of many species (e.g., psittacine birds, pigeons, raptors, and ratites). The problem is related to improper nesting conditions, keeping the birds on a smooth, slippery surface or without any lateral support, which militates against the chick standing up and bearing weight on its legs. A great and rapid increase in weight may contribute to the development of this condition together with a multiple vitamin and mineral deficiency or at least an imbalance of nutrients. The result is a unilateral or bilateral torsion of the hip or stifle joints or subluxation of the intertarsal joint.
(b) Treatment consists of fixating the legs in a normal physiologic position using adhesive tape or a partially sliced block of polyurethane foam to form a hobble. The bird should be kept in an upright position and on a pad of polyurethane foam into which it can dig its claws. Treatment can be successful if initiated at an early stage of the disease.

183 **(a)** There is a pronounced increase in bone density around the shoulder joint. No joint space can be discerned. This is almost certainly caused by ankylosis of the head of the humerus and the glenoid cavity. Also, the musculature around this joint has atrophied. This is a common result if a bird's wing has been kept strapped up for too long.
(b) A radiograph should have been made of this injury at the earliest opportunity, to ascertain the extent of damage. Then, if there were no fractures that required splinting, the wing should have been strapped with a figure-8 bandage for perhaps 3 to 4 days, after which the bandage should have been removed and the injury reassessed. Providing the primary feathers were not trailing on the ground, the bandage could be left off or replaced for a further

short period and then again reassessed. Leaving the bandage on for a prolonged period not only results in marked muscle atrophy but also reduces peripheral circulation and encourages the formation of fibrosis in injured tissue. After removal of the bandage, the bird should be encouraged to exercise the injured limb for short but regular intervals. Providing bathing facilities for a convalescent gull will help to achieve this objective.

184 (a) Because striated muscle fibers are considered to be the most important component of both the sphincter and dilator muscles of the avian pupil, movement of the pupil is to a certain degree under voluntary control and the pupillary light reflex is unreliable. The pupil responds poorly to light but actively to temperamental factors. There is no dilation of the pupil with atropine.
(b) The color of the iris depends on age, sex, and species and may be brown, black, yellow, green, red, or pale blue. This high degree of physiologic variation makes it difficult to give a judgment on abnormal coloration of the iris. However, discoloration of the iris and its atrophy may be seen after iridocyclitis, which is usually irreversible.
(c) The avian lens has a nonoptic, ringlike peripheral region termed the *annular pad,* and overall the lens is much softer than in mammals. The powers of accommodation are well developed in birds because of the prominent cramptonian muscle. A striated muscle, approximately 20 diopters, is possible.

185 (a) There is obvious multiple abscessation of both liver and spleen. The rest of the visible viscera appear normal.
(b) Milliary abscessation of the liver and spleen in birds may be caused by avian tuberculosis, *E. coli,* salmonellosis, or *Yersinia pseudotuberculosis.* In some avian families, such as those containing the owls, falcons, and cranes, specific herpesvirus infections can mimic these lesions. Herpesvirus infection in parrots (Pacheco's disease) is not quite like this.
(c) Subsequent to the gross postmortem examination, specimens should be obtained for histopathology and microbiologic culture. This particular case turned out to be one of *Y. pseudotuberculosis,* which is of common occurrence in outside aviaries during the more inclement months of the year.
(d) The infection is carried by wild birds that form flocks during the winter, allowing infection to be more easily passed from bird to bird. Also, wild birds may be more debilitated because of food shortages, the stress of young birds learning to survive, and so on. The wild bird may perch on the wire netting roof of an aviary, through which it defecates and thereby contaminates food and water bowls. Wild rodents also carry the infection and can infect food supplies. The organism is motile and can replicate outside the living animal. Many soil invertebrates can act as mechanical carriers. Consequently, once an aviary is infected, only a very thorough disinfection program is likely to eliminate the organism. All aviaries should be not only rodent proof but also covered to protect from wild birds. Aviaries also should not have soil bases.

186 (a) This bird has two fractured wings. A fractured coracoid on the left side and a fractured ulna on the right side.
(b) Because segments of the comminuted fracture of the ulna on the right side are not greatly displaced and the unfractured radius is acting as a natural splint, this side does not require surgery. The wing is best strapped to itself in the flexed position using a figure-8 bandage. The bandage is left in place for 6 to 7 days then totally removed. Regarding the left side, even comminuted or highly displaced fractures of the coracoid seldom require surgical intervention. Surgery of these fractures is complicated by a difficult approach to the fracture site

and the close proximity of the heart and major blood vessels. Taping the affected wing to the body for 3 to 4 weeks, depending on the bird's size, is usually sufficient to achieve adequate healing. Sometimes cage rest alone is sufficient if the bird is kept in a quiet environment. If the wing is taped, a nonadhesive tape, such as a self-adhesive elastic bandage, should be used because some adhesives cause damage to the plumage. Because of the protection provided by surrounding muscle masses, coracoid fractures are very rarely compound and so do not usually require antibiotics. It should be noted that a grossly displaced and healed but malaligned fracture of the coracoid can potentially cause partial obstruction of the crop or esophagus, and therefore the prognosis must always be guarded.

187 Results obtained from the disc diffusion susceptibility test are not necessarily reliable for birds because the semiquantitative classification is commonly based on plasma concentrations of antibiotics obtained from mammals. Further knowledge of the pharmacokinetics of the chosen antibiotic in the species that is to be treated is important (e.g., the half-life of doxycycline is much shorter in Amazon parrots [*Amazon* spp.] and cockatoos [*Cacatua* spp.] than in other parrots; enrofloxacin is eliminated via the kidneys more rapidly in African gray parrots [*P. erithacus*] than in Amazon parrots and cockatoos; the pharmacokinetics of chloramphenicol vary widely among bird species).
After administration of a chosen antibiotic a change from this drug to another antibiotic should be considered if no clinical response is seen within 48 hours.

188 **(a)** This cell is considered to be a monocyte. Monocytes are usually the largest and the least numerous of the leukocytes seen in avian blood smears. The cell nucleus is eccentrically positioned and usually round to oval or elongated with an indentation on one side or, in some cases, bilobed. The nuclear chromatin is finely granular to reticular and may show a few dense clumps. The basophilic cell matrix is abundant and frequently fine-grained, vacuolated, or foamy, with mostly irregular cytoplasmic borders. It may contain a dark blue central area partly surrounded by a light-staining marginal zone (hyaline mantle) adjacent to the nucleus. Next to the nuclear indentation, cytoplasm is where the reticulation is more obvious, giving a vacuolated appearance. Because of their size, monocytes are distorted more readily during the process of making dried smears than are small cells.
(b) In birds, a persistent monocytosis is commonly associated with chronic organ-reacting disease, (e.g., a septic form of chlamydiosis, Pacheco's disease), tissue necrosis, and granuloma formation—notably *Mycobacterium avium* infections, salmonellosis, yersiniosis, and fungal infections. According to some authors, monocytosis is noted in the recovery phase of bacterial or chlamydial infections and in the acute phase of certain diseases. Absence of nuclear indentation, excess cytoplasm, and vacuolation might be seen in cases of bacterial or fungal infection.

189 **(a)** Generally a single broken or missing feather does not have much influence on flight capability.
(b) Single missing flight feathers are physiologically often seen during molt until the new feather grows to occupy the position of the molted feather.
(c) Normally such single defects can easily be compensated for, but there is a very slight risk that the neighboring feathers may be damaged or broken during flight because of increased mechanical stress as a result of interruption of the continuity of feather pattern. To prevent this the broken section of feather can be replaced by a process known as *imping* (from the Latin *impono*). This is carried out by using a wooden, bamboo peg or metal needle as a guide inserted into the feather shaft of the broken feather, with the opposing end

inserted into the shaft of the replacement feather. Both the remaining section of feather and the replacement end sections are cut obliquely at the same angle and then glued together, preferably with an epoxy resin glue. The vane of the repaired feather must precisely overlap the neighboring feathers in the same manner as its predecessor. It is best to use feathers from a previous molt from the same species because replacement feathers must be of the same size and have the same mechanical characteristics (i.e., strength and flexibility, which vary among species depending of mode of flight) as the original feather.

190 (a) A definitive diagnosis can only be made after microbiologic and other laboratory tests. In this bird, *Aspergillus* spp. and *Mucor* spp. were isolated from this lesion and were assumed to be the primary pathogens. However, if there were signs of a feather dystrophy, then viral psittacine beak and feather syndrome should be considered in the differential diagnoses. Hypovitaminosis A also seems to play an important role in the susceptibility of the beak to mycotic infection.
(b) Affected birds respond well to a treatment consisting of repeated injections of vitamin A (7500 IU/kg body weight every 3 to 7 days for a maximum of six doses; overdosage is toxic producing skeletal abnormalities). These injections should be combined with the daily topical application of enilconazole diluted 1:5 in water until the defect is healed, which may take some weeks.

191 Slight movement blur is apparent. The bird's legs should be pulled caudally as far as possible to avoid superimposition of the legs on the body.
The bird has an obvious healed fracture of the left tibiotarsus. It is possible that this bird was treated in the past by some unknown person and then released back into its wild habitat. However, there is no sign of any identification ring or even a microchip, which would have been expected had the bird been treated in a rehabilitation centre. On the other hand it is quite possible the bone may have healed while the bird remained in the wild. Similar cases have been documented. The muscle mass over the affected leg is marginally smaller than on the other side so that the bird might still be slightly lame.
The ventriculus occupying the coelom is filled with the skeletal remains of the bird's prey, indicating the bird has recently fed and the undigested food particles of prey skeleton and so on have not yet been ejected as a pellet. It would have been wiser in the circumstances to have starved this bird for 24 hours before radiography. Also, because this is a road accident case, a radiograph should have been made of the head.

192 (a) Several avian species often kept as pet birds have no external sexual characteristics, that is, they are sexually monomorphic.
The following two main methods are commonly used for sex differentiation:
• Blood collection, usually by clipping a toenail and collecting the blood in a capillary tube, for examination of the DNA in a specialized laboratory. This noninvasive procedure can be used at a very early stage. Methods for collecting DNA for sexing from feather samples are now also being developed and are even less invasive.
• Surgical sexing can be performed by laparoscopy. Direct visualization by laparoscopy provides the advantage of allowing evaluation of reproductive organs with special regard to size and activity, as well as allowing inspection of other intraabdominal structures. Its main disadvantages are that it is invasive and there is an anesthetic risk.
(b) The bird on the left has a feather dysplasia over its ventral body surface. At the same time a blood examination for DNA sexing is performed, another DNA check for psittacine beak and feather disease should be recommended.

Answers

193 (a) Distinct enlargement of the proventriculus is visible in this radiograph. One of the possible diseases with such clinical signs and radiographic findings is proventricular dilation syndrome (see the answer to Fig. 170). This is a chronic disease of the digestive system that, apart from signs of alimentary dysfunction, can occasionally result in signs of CNS disease. The incubation period can be as long as 2 years, and mortality among affected birds is 100%.
(b) Other diseases exhibiting similar clinical signs may be bacterial or mycotic (e.g., *Candida* spp.) infection, infestation with parasites (especially tape worms but also *Ascaridia* spp.). Neoplasms should also be considered. Confirmation of diagnosis of psittacine proventricular dilation syndrome has been attempted using biopsy of the proventriculus or crop, but this does not provide 100% confirmation. It is important to rule out any differential diagnosis.

194 (a) This is a multiple fracture of the humerus.
(b) Correct resolution of this lesion will require rigid fixation of the fracture site. Intramedullary pinning as the only means of fixation does not provide sufficient rotational stability. Moreover, the relatively large diameter of the pin required to fill the medullary cavity places a disproportionate amount of weight on the injured tissues, not only the bone but also adjacent traumatized soft tissue, and also disrupts the internal trabeculae of the bone. The latter are part of the integral strength of the bone, which undergoes up to 70 degrees of rotational torque during flight.
Using external fixation alone, such as a figure-8 bandage, will not provide sufficient stability to keep the two end segments of the bone in alignment. Bone plates are not practical in a bird of this size, because the thin cortex of the bone does not provide a sufficiently good bed for the screws. Probably the best solution is to use a Kirschner type of splint with four Kirschner pins, two in the proximal segment and two in the distal segment, anchored externally with epoxy glue, after transfixing plastic tube, which is stiffened and held straight by one or more Kirschner-Ehmer wires. This now-rigid plastic tube runs parallel to the bone. Other methods, such as the Harrison/Doyle impaction technique or an intramedullary peg and figure-8 wiring, have also have been used. Conservative therapy is difficult in treating humeral fractures and is limited to proximal fractures of this bone, because the strong muscles of the wing (M. biceps brachii, M. triceps brachii, and M. brachialis) go into spasm, pulling the two ends of the bone together and causing the segments at the fracture site to override.
Whatever method of fixation is employed, the small detached middle section of bone is best removed, otherwise it is likely to become a sequestrum. It can be crushed into small granules and deposited around the fracture site to help promote mineralization of this area by the interaction of osteoclasts and osteoblasts.
(c) Possible infection of the air sac system should always be considered because of the extrathoracic diverticula extension of the clavicular air sac into the medullary cavity of the humerus. Regarding convalescence, because of all bird's high rates of metabolism, food intake should occur at least every 24 hours, otherwise force-feeding by gavage tube must begin. The natural prey of sparrowhawks are small wild birds. Laboratory mice and surplus hatchery chicks may not be recognized as food by this raptor. Sparrowhawks are highly nervous birds that are easily stressed in captivity and should therefore be kept in a quiet environment with as little handling and disturbance as possible.

195 (a) These are the eggs of so-called biting lice and are glued to the feather shafts.
(b) These parasitic invertebrates, almost entirely confined to birds, belong to the order Mallophaga, whereas the "true" lice are taxonomically placed in the order Anoplura. Mallophaga are host-specific. Most of them feed on feathers and cell debris from the kera-

tinized layer of epidermis. Some species of the suborder Amblycera suck blood by chewing the growing feather quill. The prepatent period is 3 to 5 weeks, and the adult parasites' life span is 2 to 3 months. The pathogenicity of mallophagans is usually low and results mainly in pruritus, restlessness, and damaged plumage. Bloodsucking genera may cause skin disorders as well as anemia and death in very young birds. Healthy birds usually keep these parasites under control by constant grooming, and therefore massive infestation as in the case illustrated may hint at other underlying problems.
(c) Affected birds may be treated by the application of powders or sprays containing organophosphates, pyrethrum, or carbaryl. This therapy does not affect the parasites' eggs, and, because the adults cannot survive longer than 14 days when isolated from the host, treatment should be repeated after 2 to 3 weeks.

196 (a) The great vessels of the heart, the brachiocephalic trunk, and the aorta look somewhat thickened with a faint yellowish tinge. Although the vessels are not irregularly shaped, as is often the case, these signs indicate a tentative diagnosis of atherosclerosis.
(b) This would be confirmed by histopathology.

197 (a) These are tawny owls *(Strix aluco)*. They are primarily woodland owls and range over much of Eurasia as far as Burma, the Himalayas, and China and also are found in northwest Africa. These are all young fledglings that still have some of their immature plumage and have not completely lost all of their down feathering (particularly noticeable over the head).
(b) These young owls are approximately 30 days old.
(c) At this age, tawny owls leave the nest and attempt to fly, often landing on the ground and then climbing up the surrounding trees to repeat the process. During this time they gain flying ability, familiarize themselves with their surroundings, and learn to hunt, but continue to be fed and cared for by the parent birds until they are about 4 months old.
(d) If these immature birds are returned within 24 hours to the site where they were found, the parent birds will continue to look after them.

198 (a) On palpation the swelling feels soft and balloonlike. Insertion of a hypodermic needle into the point of greatest distension results in immediate collapse of the inflated area. If in doubt, radiography may help to confirm the diagnosis.
(b) The precise extent of the single median clavicular air sac (present in most species of birds, except loons or divers [*Gaviidae*]) varies with the taxonomy. In some groups of birds (e.g., song birds) the clavicular air sac fuses with the two cranial thoracic sacs. In all species, however, it occupies the thoracic inlet, sending diverticulae extending around the heart and major blood vessels and along the sternum. Extrathoracic diverticulae penetrate between the muscles and bones surrounding the thoracic inlet and also extend into the medullary cavities of some of the bones.
(c) Although insertion of a hypodermic needle results in temporary deflation, a fistula (best created using radiosurgery) is necessary for a more permanent collapse of the swelling. This will take pressure off the primary wound responsible for the original rupture of the air sac, giving the lesion a chance to heal.

199 (a) The following are the differential diagnoses:
• A neoplasm, the exact nature of which can only be determined by histopathology. Adenomas and adenocarcinomas of the uropygial gland are not uncommon, particularly in budgerigars. Other neoplasms, such as squamous cell carcinomas, also occur.

• Impaction of the uropygial gland. Because the gland is a bilobed structure, it is possible in this particular case that only one lobe (the left) is impacted.
• Abscessation of the uropygial gland that may be secondary to impaction. Diagnosis can be confirmed not only by histopathology but by cytology and microbiologic culture of an aspirate.
(b) In this case surgical excision of the complete lesion is the simplest solution after ligation of the pedicle. If such a lesion is not so pendulous, prior treatment with hot, moist compresses may relieve an impacted or abscessated gland and possibly should be followed with an incision of the dorsal surface and expression of the contents. During surgery care must be taken not to damage the follicles of the rectrices.

200 (a) On the left side of the posterior choanal opening in the region of the medial palatine salivary glands occurs a cream-colored "necrotic" area.
(b) The following are the differential diagnoses are:
• *Capillaria* infestation
• *Candida* spp. infection
• *Trichomonas* spp. infection
• Herpesvirus infection
• Bacterial infection, which may be primary or secondary to any of the above

201 (a) This is a case of gross impaction of the cloaca, primarily with urate crystals. The bird has been straining to pass this impaction, as is evident from the prolapsed and dilated cloacal mucus membrane and expanded vent. The feathering around the vent is unnaturally contaminated with concreted urates, indicating that this bird was not passing normal feces before the impaction.
(b) The precise etiology of cloacal impaction is not always easy to determine. It may occur after a cloacitis, from an ingested foreign body (a sliver of wood may have passed uneventfully through a psittacine's alimentary until becoming wedged in the cloaca), or as the result of a retained egg. A large cloacal neoplasm together with secondary infection may result in cloacal impaction, as might prolonged dehydration.

202 (a) This is a case of severe crop burning, which in a bird of this age may not be the result of a single instance of crop burn (i.e., food given once in excess of 48° C [120° F]) but is more likely due to the food being given a little too hot over a prolonged period (i.e., 46° C [115° F]).
(b) The temperature of food should be between 38° to 40° C (101° to 104° F). Often the bird will quite happily take food that is too hot and show no signs of discomfort. The owner may not be aware of the problem until the abnormal swelling is noticed or the bird feels wet around the crop area and food is noticed on the outside of the swelling, the necrotic skin having ruptured and formed a fistula. In such a case the skin will have become adherent to the underlying crop. In a case such as the one illustrated it is probably wiser to leave the lesion alone for 10 days to allow initial conservative treatment, (i.e., administering antibiotics), leaving the wound to granulate and giving smaller but more frequent feeds. Should the fistula enlarge greatly and the whole area break down, a pharyngostomy tube reaching into the proventriculus must be inserted and the separated and débrided crop and skin defects repaired over the underlying tube. If the healthy tissues cannot be brought together, the wound should be covered with a hydrophilic dressing that can be lightly sutured in place.

203 From the presence of medullary bone in the coracoids, the clavicles, the scapulae, the radii, the ulnas, the femurs, and the tibiotarsal bones it must be assumed this bird is in the egg-laying phase of its reproductive cycle. However, there is no sign of an egg, although the gizzard with its retained grit has been displaced cranially and to the left. This could be due to the presence of a retained soft-shelled egg. The whole coelumic area looks rather "cloudy," and there is little differentiation between the heart and liver shadows. This may indicate a degree of air sacculitis and peritonitis, with an enlarged liver. There are signs of retained urate concretions in the cloaca, which may be due to dehydration.

On postmortem examination this bird had an advanced egg peritonitis, air sacculitis, and gross fibrinous adhesions to the viscera. Also, there was a retained soft-shelled egg in the oviduct and fatty infiltration of the liver. Abscessation was present in the caudal aspects of both lungs.

204 **(a)** A midshaft erosion of the lateral cortex of the tarsometatarsus has occurred, probably as a result of pressure necrosis and secondary infection caused by a metal closed identification ring.
(b) Generally, a numbered ring is placed over the foot of a young fledgling. At this age, this is a fairly easy procedure because the foot is supple and the small foot can be passed through the relatively large ring. Usually, slightly smaller rings are used for male birds in contrast to the somewhat larger rings used for female chicks. However, it is not always easy to know the sex of the birds at 10 or 11 days of age, and often a male ring is placed on one foot and a female ring is placed on the other foot, with the intention being to remove the inappropriate ring at a later date. Sometimes removal is forgotten, and a bird, usually a female, is left with a ring which is too small for it. The ring becomes tight, does not rotate around the shank freely, and initiates an inflammatory reaction in the underlying scales. In response, the scales become hypertrophied, the ring becomes embedded in the enlarged dermal tissue, and ulceration commences.
(c) The area around the margins of the lesion show an increase in bone density and there is some evidence of a periosteal reaction, indicating that this lesion must be a minimum of 21 days old.
(d) The following points should be considered in the surgical procedure for treatment:
• The lesion must be thoroughly cleansed and curetted to encourage new bone growth. Swabs should be taken for microbiologic culture.
• Keeping this lesion in only an external splint may result in the flexor tendons becoming trapped in callus.
• The most effective surgical method of holding the lesion firmly in position while it heals is by placement of four full-length pins (of arthrodesis or Kirschner wires), two placed proximal to the lesion and two distal to the lesion and placed from the lateral to medial sides. The pins should be passed through two lengths of plastic tubing, one on the medial aspect and one on the lateral aspect and running parallel to the diaphysis of the bone. After positioning, the pins are held rigidly in tubes filled with methylmethacrylate, epoxy resin glue, or dental acrylic. Because the proximal part of this bone in the goshawk is rather flattened craniocaudally, care must be taken to ensure that the pins do not slip off the cortex and damage the flexor and extensor tendons, which run on the cranial and caudal aspects of the bone. It should also be noted that the flexor tendons run in a groove on the caudal aspect of the bone. When placing the pins, care should be taken to avoid the medially placed flexor tendon of insertion of the hallux (i.e., the first digit).

205 **(a)** This cell is considered to be a (large) lymphocyte compared with other leukocytes. Lymphocytes are relatively small (6 to 12 μm in diameter), spherical cells containing a scarce, pale blue, mostly homogenous cytoplasm that may contains several basophilic (but rarely azurophilic) granules. Vacuoles, if present at all, are very small and round. The nucleus is usually round and centrally located. However the regular rounded outline of the lymphocyte may frequently be broken by pseudopodial projections. According to size, lymphocytes are arbitrarily classified into three groups. The amount of cytoplasm varies from a narrow band surrounding the nucleus in small lymphocytes to a moderately wide band in medium and large lymphocytes.

(b) Lymphocytes are sensitive to a heavy-handed technique during slide preparation and are often squashed, making cells appear to have more cytoplasm than is actually the case. When this is encountered (or suspected) it is best to use nuclear characteristics aided by cytoplasmic coloration as a method of identification and differentiation from other cell types. Because lymphocytes often throw out blebs of cytoplasm (thus making it difficult to judge total cell size), this assessment of cell size also applies to the classification of intact cells and the differentiation between lymphocytes and monocytes. Although the two types of cells are not functionally related, their cell morphology on stained smears can be very similar. According to some authors, it is easiest to speak of a lymphocyte/monocyte continuum, because there are many intermediate forms that are difficult to classify and this problem is increased by inter bird species diversity. Indentation of the nucleus, although not common in lymphocytes, is often given as a reliable criterion for differentiation. Usually any depression is not deep and, as in this case, the margins curve inward to a base with a sharp angle rather than forming a depression with a rounded base as often occurs in monocytes.

(c) Under normal conditions, lymphocytes are often the most numerous leukocytes found in the peripheral blood of pet birds. Said to be in a resting state, the small lymphocyte is the size most commonly encountered. In contrast to the total white cell and heterophil counts, species variation in lymphocytes is far less common.

(d) Regarding abnormal erythrocytes, these show hemolysis resulting from osmotic damage (in this case rain drops on the smear before fixation). Hemolysis (as well as postmortem changes) may interfere with staining characteristics, resulting in the appearance of mature erythrocytes similar to reticulocytes; therefore cytologic diagnosis should be confirmed by anamnestic and clinical findings. Additional data (i.e., packed cell volume, hemoglobin concentration, and total protein content of serum or plasma) are of particular importance.

206 The following are two commonly used methods of catching large psittacines:
• Wearing a thick protective glove will make catching the bird easier. The disadvantage of this method is that the bird can clearly visualize and attack the person's hand. Many birds that have been quarantined are familiar with this method and become aggressive as soon as the glove is seen.
• A better method is to use a hand towel laid over the spread fingers of the hand. Many birds do not identify the approaching object with a catching hand and are less likely to attack and bite the handler. One should attempt to quickly grasp and fixate the bird's head in the cheek region (mandibular joints) or encircle the neck with thumb and forefinger. Care should be taken to hold the wings close to the handler's body to prevent fractures or injuries to the wings. Often the hanging ends of the towel can be quickly wrapped around the bird to restrain wings and feet. If practical, it is usually easier to remove the base of the cage, tip the cage on its side, and approach the bird through the bottom opening. In very nervous or difficult birds it may be easier to catch the bird in a dark room using only the light from a blue-filtered flashlight. Many birds do not see well in blue light.

207 (a) Digits I and III show erythema. An additional edematous swelling is visible on the second digit and on the plantar surface of the foot. Furthermore, a dark discoloration can be seen on the second pad of digit II, and the skin of the leg and the skin covering the tarsometatarsal region show epidermal defects.

187

(b) These findings suggest a second-degree burn that likely resulted from electrocution. This condition is commonly caused by contact of the extremities with the poles of medium- to high-voltage power lines (not the large pylons, as seen in the United Kingdom [the electrical insulators are spaced too far apart]). A considerable number of affected birds die from the trauma following a fall to the ground.

(c) Examination of electrocuted birds should include inspection of the plumage for further burn marks, which can be very small and indistinct, palpation and radiographic examination for fractures, and cardiologic examination. Any evidence of shock also should be taken into account. Birds injured during the summer months should be checked for myiasis.

208 First, it is necessary to differentiate between a flaccid paralysis, which is of neurogenic origin, and a lameness caused by pain. The latter may be caused by fractures, arthritis, or soft tissue damage (sprain, abscess, etc.) to the locomotor system, and a thorough visual and palpation examination of the affected limb will usually reveal the underlying problem. With a unilateral paralysis, it is essential to take radiographs. Intraabdominal space-occupying lesions, especially those of renal and gonadal origin can cause lameness because of their close association with the lumbosacral plexus and potential compression of the ischiadic nerve.

209 **(a)** A hypocalcemia has been found to produce the clinical signs that often will show the bird to be hyperesthetic (hypersensitive). Among psittacines, the gray parrot seems particularly prone to this problem, but the entire etiology remains unclear. The disease process is commonly induced by a calcium or vitamin D_3 deficiency (i.e., feeding only seed), but only a few birds on a low-calcium diet will develop the symptoms. A virus infection of the parathyroid gland has been suggested, and oxytetracycline medication by chelating serum calcium may precipitate a subclinical condition. Serum blood level testing for calcium may be an indicator but is not a reliable method to establish a definitive diagnosis. This is because clinical signs may occur, even when serum calcium levels are still within the normal range. In contrast to this, many birds with low blood calcium levels are asymptomatic.

(b) Affected birds respond well to slow intravenous injections of calcium gluconate or calcium borogluconate (50 to 100 mg/kg body weight) or intramuscular injections of 5 to 10 mg/kg. The diet should be changed, or a calcium and vitamin D_3 supplement should be added, so that a total amount of 0.3% calcium and 2000 IU of vitamin D_3 is added per kilogram of food.

210 **(a)** The Amazon parrot (*Amazona* spp.) would be better restrained using a towel. However, placing a plastic syringe of adequate size between upper and lower beak is a perfectly proper method of maintaining the oral cavity open but only provides limited access. It is suitable when taking swabs from the oropharynx and crop, or for crop washings, to prevent the bird biting the swab or tube. Nevertheless, visual examination of this area is limited. For this purpose it is better to use two pieces of gauze (or several thicknesses in the case of large birds with powerful, sharp-edged beaks) held between fingers and thumb of each hand, or the layers of gauze can be hooked to upper and lower beak and pulled apart (not always easy).

(b) Alternatively, a canine auriscope gives reasonable but still limited access. Metal speculae of varying sizes are available for this purpose. Psittacines apart, the shape and size of the beak (even in some raptors, such as the goshawk [*Accipiter gentilis gentilis*]) will permit a digital exploration even as far as the crop. When using a speculum of any sort, care must be taken not to damage the oral mucosa or edges of the beak.

211 (a) There are indications of subchondral bone lysis. The intercondylar space is eroded, and there is an extensive periostitis with signs of epiphyte formation. All of this is a result of a septic arthritis. If samples are obtained by aspiration for microbiologic culture, the offending pathogen may sometimes be identified. However, this may only be a secondary invader. If sterile, this could be due to salmonellosis.
(b) The most likely predisposing factors in the domestic goose are obesity and the bird having been kept on an unsuitable substrate. The domestic goose originally evolved from the eastern greylag goose, which is an active flier that inhabits areas of soft marshy ground, peat moss, and the seashore. Domestic backyard geese are often kept on small, dried out paddocks with little or no water for bathing.
(c) Therapeutically suitable antibiotics may be indicated, and a nonsteroidal antiinflammatory drug such as ketoprofen (1 mg/kg body weight IM once daily for 1 to 10 days) may give some temporary relief. In geese, these lesions are often caused by salmonellosis. However, whether this is the direct etiology or not, surgery is an alternative method of treating such lesions. The diseased bone and cartilage are removed to create an arthrodesis or possibly a pseudo joint.
(d) Long-term results are often good.

212 Bone was carefully removed with a dental burr from the proximolateral surface of the ulna for a distance of approximately 1 cm. The pin was exposed and then carefully eased out of the medullary cavity. Prophylactic antibiotic cover was given using clindamycin (10 mg/kg body weight q8-12h).

213 The chicks of altricial species, such as psittacines, are helpless at hatch, naked, and unable to thermoregulate. The nestling's age and the amount of feathering determine the optimal ambient temperature. At hatch, this temperature should be 33° to 37° C (92° to 94° F), which, over the course of the next few weeks when the chick becomes fully feathered, may be reduced to 24° to 32° C (75° to 87° F). The chick's behavior and appearance will indicate if it is too hot or too cold. Single chicks usually require a somewhat higher temperature than three or four chicks reared together, when the total body mass is increased.
Humidity should be such that it will prevent the chick from drying out and dehydrating or, if too moist, from adhering to the inner shell membrane. For tropical species, humidity should be about 50% to 60%, but this will vary slightly according to the habitat of origin of the species. Some species originate from relatively dry lowland areas.
If a chick is not reared at the optimal temperature and humidity, its growth will be retarded and it is liable to develop crop emptying problems.
Most of the exact nutritional requirements of psittacine hatchlings are not well documented and are largely based on the experience of the individual bird breeder.

214 (a) This chick is showing signs of splayed leg syndrome. The left hip joint is possibly affected, and on the right side probably both the hip and stifle joints are affected. There is also a suspicion of valgus deformity of the left intertarsal joint. All of these can be confirmed by radiography.
(b) All of these problems are the result of multifactorial malnutrition, principally hypovitaminosis vitamin D_3 and low calcium, and a high protein and energy intake. These conditions result in a rapidly growing, relatively heavy chick with insufficiently strong skeletal structures to support it. A chick raised on a slippery work surface (e.g., a surface covered with a laminate product or a plastic tub for cleanliness) is liable to predisposing trauma. A subclinical polyomavirus infection has also been suggested.

(c) Treatment consists of hobbling the legs in some manner, such as with adhesive tape or placing the legs in the correct alignment in slits cut in a block of expanded polyurethane foam and taping this together. In any case, supporting the chick, wedged with paper towel, in the upright position in a tub is essential. Placing a deep mat of expanded polyurethane foam in the depth of the supporting tub helps the chick to grip and encourages movement of the claws. A variation of this method is to use sections of plumbers' polyurethane pipe wrap slit across the diameter and laid side by side in the bottom of a box or tube. Obviously, for hygienic purposes this should be changed frequently, but it does enable the chick to dig into the surface with its claws. Hobbles should be adjusted every 3 to 4 days. The diet must be suitably adjusted. For very mild cases, placing the bird in a deep cup may work. Correction of the valgus deformity may have to wait until the bone is fully ossified, when a Kirschner splinting technique may be used.

215 (a) This bird is a cassowary. It is a member of the double-wattled species (*Casuarius casuarius*).
(b) There are three species in the genus, all of which come from Australasia. This particular species originates from the rain forests of Papua New Guinea and northeastern Australia.
(c) These powerful birds can be very aggressive; this is the most dangerous bird a veterinarian is ever likely to handle. The bird can kick forward and, unlike the ostrich, backward and swing out sideways. The foot is tridactyl, with the middle digit (i.e., the third digit) possessing a lethal daggerlike claw. When cornered, these birds roll onto their backs and flail out with the upturned feet. They are also capable of jumping. No attempt should be made to examine the conscious bird's legs or feet. The bird should be persuaded to enter a crush with solid wooden sides approximately 4 feet (1.2 m) long with sides 4 feet high. These stocks should be about 2 feet wide at the front, with the sides hinged so that they can be folded and held firmly against the entrapped bird. A removable bar is positioned to stop the bird retreating out of the crush. A strong strap should be positioned across the top. The sides have a 9- to 10-inch (22- to 25-cm) gap at the bottom for the splayed feet of the bird. After securing the crush, an attempt should be made to place a hood (made of cloth, such as a sweatshirt) on the bird. However, the bird may not tolerate this. If achieved, hooding will make the bird more manageable. Working quietly in a dimmed light makes for less troublesome handling. The bird should be anaesthetized with an intravenous injection of ketamine hydrochloride (5 to 10 mg/kg body weight) and xylazine (1 mg/kg body weight) or etorphine (0.01 mg/kg body weight). Intramuscular diazepam alone is unlikely to provide sufficient sedation, and induction with isoflurane tends to be prolonged. Because it may be difficult to use the muscle of the legs for injection, the muscle on either side of the spine can be used.

216 The microbiologic culture of swabs taken from a bird's oral or nasal cavity may reveal microorganisms that are not necessarily the primary etiologic agents of disease. Often, fungal agents are secondary contaminants and result from problems of hygiene within a flock (e.g., a high degree of fungal contamination of the food supply). On the other hand, *Aspergillus* spp. and *Penicillium* spp. are also potential pathogens in psittacines, particularly if they are found in large numbers in the sample and if they are in almost pure culture combined with the presence of clinical signs (e.g., respiratory symptoms).

217 (a) Radiography and possibly ultrasonography may reveal the exact relationship of this structure to the normal anatomic structures of the neck. Ultrasonography particularly may reveal whether this abnormal structure is of uniform density. Barium contrast will reveal whether this swelling involves the esophagus. If there is any suspicion that ulceration of the esophagus has occurred through a penetrating foreign body (e.g., a needle or spicule of wood), endoscopy may help.

(b) Apart from an abscess or neoplasm, which are possible etiologies, this almost spherical swelling measuring 7.5 cm when eventually dissected out was found to be an organized hematoma. Bleeding had occurred on at least three separate occasions because the lesion had an onion-skin structure.

218 (a) The plumage on the head and neck has reasonably normal pigmentation for this species. However, the dark, dull feathering of most of the minor and some of the medium coverts indicates old, worn, and frayed feathering retained well beyond its normal molting period. There are also suspicions of worn areas on some of the major coverts and on tail feathers.
The dark red plumage of the back is normal for the species, but the yellow and orange of some of the medium and major coverts and of some of the primary feathers is abnormal, as is the patch of pink on one vane of a primary feather. It is suggested that this yellow-orange-pink coloring is possibly caused by changes in the keratin structure of the feather, so that the normal blue element of the feather coloring caused by the scattering of blue light does not take place. In these circumstances the yellow pigment (derived from plant carotenoids) becomes dominant; the normal green color results from a combination with blue (structurally produced light and yellow pigment). It is to be noted that there are present some normal green major coverts and some normal green primary and tail feathers. There is no evidence of fret or hunger marks or evidence of self-mutilation.
(b) All of this indicates that this bird has not been molting regularly for some time, and that some change has abruptly occurred in its normal metabolism, resulting in the production of abnormally colored feathers.
(c) Therapy included the use of thyroid hormone (liothyronine sodium 20 μg/kg body weight q24h) for 5 days only to induce molt. The use of thyroid hormone is equivocal, and testosterone or progesterone may be better. The thyroid hormone was supplemented with iodine (diluted Lugol's iodine in the drinking water) and gradual introduction of a commercial pelleted diet to make sure all the necessary nutrients in the diet were being provided. A routine was suggested to gradually increase the bird's daily exercise.

219 (a) Some congenital defects occur in birds as genetic cataracts. Genetic cataracts are seen especially in macaws and canaries. Cataracts may also be seen as juvenile, senile, or traumatic types. The grade of cloudiness of the lens may vary; the alteration may be either diffuse or focal.
(b) Senile cataracts may occur in a variety of avian species, such as old parrots, canaries, and even raptors, although documented senile cataracts are rarely seen in free-living wild birds. The exact pathogenesis of senile cataract formation is unknown. Besides the age of the bird, nutrition, hormonal balance, and constitution (i.e., overall general fitness) are all thought to play a role in the etiology of the disease.
Bacterial infection of the iris, choroidea, and ciliary body may lead to uveitis and secondary cataract formation. Cataract resulting from infection may occur bilaterally and lead to the formation of glaucoma. A cataract together with a secondary glaucoma may also be due to traumatic injury.
(c) Because the incidence of primary cataracts in birds is rare and therefore not well documented, the justification for the surgical removal of the avian cataractous lens is questionable. Prior investigation may be required to prove the normal function of the retina by electroretinography. The loss of visual accommodation after removal of the lens must be considered, although some of these birds have been used in falconry displays, particularly if only one eye is involved.

Self-assessment picture tests
Avian Medicine

220 (a) A, This is an advanced interstitial keratitis with almost complete loss of transparency, except for some of the extreme perimeter. There is the suspicion of a corneal ulcer in the center of the lesion, and there are signs of a keratoconus caused by weakening of the corneal structure. There is some superficial vascularization extending from the 7 to 8 o'clock position across the dorsal surface of the cornea.

(b) This lesion is almost certainly the end result of a traumatic incident that did not receive adequate initial treatment.

(c) Obtain swabs for microbiologic culture of secondary contaminating pathogens. Then suture the eyelids together with two horizontal mattress sutures. This is better than using the third eyelid as a corneal bandage, because muscular action might pull the sutures through. This first-aid measure is necessary because of the keratoconus and the danger of collapse of the globe of the eye. To improve chances of epithelialization of the cornea the enervated tissue on the surface of the lesion must be removed using a sterile dry cotton bud or by performing a punctate or grit keratotomy. After this, the eyelids should remain sutured for a minimum of 7 to 10 days. Strict eye hygiene and the use of appropriate antibiotics are necessary.

Customized eye bandages made of a hydrated collagen shield (rather like human contact lenses) can be tried, but successful use is not easy. The artificial bandage must have the correct curvature to fit the globe exactly, and keeping the lens in place is difficult because of constant movement of the third eyelid. **B** demonstrates this eye with an eye shield in place. The dark green area in the 7 o'clock position, below the reflection of the flash highlight, is the marker incorporated in the artificial eye bandage.

221 (a) There is a fracture of the right third and fourth metacarpal bones. There is no evidence of the ulna or radial carpal joints being involved, but there is a suspicion of subluxation of the alula digit. There is some congestion of the soft tissues adjacent to this area.

(b) Surgical repair using Kirshner wires attached to an external fixator is not practical in a bird of relatively small size. The objective may be achieved, but there is a grave risk of shattering the small bones and involving the neighboring joints, thereby making the situation worse. A figure-8 bandage is simple and will encourage healing of the bone but does not allow movement of the joints or muscles, and residual and permanent stiffness may result. A method used many times with success by one author is to fold a small piece of radiographic film over the leading edge of the wing just around the fracture site. This is sutured in position with three sutures placed through the film and between the shafts of the metacarpal primary feathers just caudal to where these emerge from the skin. Care must be taken to avoid the metacarpal blood vessels. This splint is lightweight and makes use of the natural splint provided by the shafts of the primary feathers anchored directly to the bone. It also allows some restricted movement of the joints so that there is less chance of unwanted fibrosis developing.

(c) The prognosis in most of these cases is good, and many similar birds have been eventually released back into their wild habitat.

222 (a) There is a well-healed fracture site in the distal third of one tibiotarsus and a suspicion of osteoarthritis of the stifle joint of the same leg. The muscle masses surrounding the tibiotarsus of both legs look very similar, indicating the bird is still using the affected leg. The fine lines in these muscle masses are due to normal ossification of the tendons.

(b) The large spherical mass of localized areas of radiodensity within the abdomen are due to the undigested skeletal elements of the bird's prey. These will be squeezed together by the ventriculus (normally within 24 hours) and then ejected as a pellet (falconer's casting).

223 **(a)** There are many different causes for upper respiratory tract symptoms in psittacine birds. These include bacterial, mycotic, or viral agents; foreign bodies; allergies; or exposure to air pollutants (e.g., possibly heavy cigarette smoke). One infectious disease in psittacines, which is a potential zoonosis, is caused by *Chlamydia psittaci* (psittacosis). Clinical signs in birds are mostly characterized by dyspnea, sneezing, conjunctivitis, sinusitis, and watery feces. In some cases CNS signs, such as torticollis, tremor, and seizures can be observed.
(b) Swabs, preferably taken (in special transport media) from the eye, pharynx, and cloaca, subjected to various laboratory tests are necessary to confirm the diagnosis.
(c) The owner should always be informed of the risk of human infection and the clinical signs of the disease in humans. These are typically flulike, with fever, headache, and respiratory symptoms; these are in fact clinical signs of a human atypical pneumonia. CNS signs and cardiac problems may also develop in advanced human cases. Pregnant women have the risk of abortion. Despite adequate and appropriate treatment the mortality rate in infected human cases is approximately 1%. Chlamydiosis is a notifiable disease in many countries, including the United Kingdom and the United States.

224 **(a)** This is the macrogametocyte of a *Leucocytozoon* sp. organism parasitizing a blood cell, which can no longer be identified because the infected cell has been greatly distorted. The remains of the host cell nucleus are seen as a long, thin band lying along the upper edge of the cell. Parasitized cells often exhibit tapering ends. The spectrum of parasitized blood cells hitherto identified comprises macrophages, leukocytes, erythrocytes, and erythroblasts. Regardless of the type of parasitized cell, pigment granules are not present. Macrogametocytes stain dark blue; whereas microgametocytes stain pale blue.
(b) The pathogenicity within a single avian species appears to vary depending on host age, breed, degree of domestication, and population density. Most species of *Leucocytozoon* sp. are relatively benign, whereas others are highly pathogenic and have been documented as causing localized epizootics in Canada geese and other wild waterfowl. Clinical signs include ruffled feathers, listlessness, anorexia, polydipsia, somnolence (occasionally the reverse), water eye discharge, dyspnea, hemoptysis, and convulsions together with ataxia just before death. There may also be green diarrheic feces.
Gametocytes might not be seen in peripheral blood circulation in lethal infections in cases of peracute infection.
The pathogenicity of the parasite appears to be related to the presence or absence of disintegrating megaloschizonts. These may be encapsulated by fibrosis, eventually becoming necrotic and calcified. In heavy infection, multiple large creamy-white lesions can be found in skeletal muscle, heart, liver, spleen, brain, and gizzard. There may also be a severe anemia and eventual hemosiderosis. Circulating gametocytes may block lung capillaries, cause pneumonia and edema of the lungs. The clinical course of the infection may be influenced by concomitant infection.

225 **(a)** The bird should preferably be hooded to make it more manageable. However, this may not be possible because the bird is not used to this method of restraint or the falconer is reluctant to carry this out on this particular bird. In any case the bird should be held on the fist with the jesses pulled down tight between the fingers of the gloved hand. A second handler then quickly grasps the bird around the shoulders and flexed carpal joints with a towel draped over his or her two outspread hands. At the same time the falconer, with his or her free hand, firmly grasps the two legs around the tarsometatarsals, placing a finger between each leg. The bird is then gently lowered onto its back on a padded surface (folded blanket, cushion, etc.). The towel holding the wings can be firmly wrapped around the bird to prevent it struggling. However, both handlers should still keep a firm hold on the bird. With the bird thus restrained, the hood if present can be removed and the eye of the conscious bird examined in more detail. Alternatively, the bird can be anesthetized (preferably with isoflurane) for examination. Initially a biopsy or cytologic sample could be obtained, but with such a lesion it is probably better to remove the whole tumor to save having to anesthetize the bird a second time.

(b) Any sort of epithelial neoplasm, including papillomata, fibrosarcomata, lymphoreticular neoplasms, or squamous cell carcinomata, as well as a variety of basal cell tumors, have the potential for affecting this area. Alternatively, the lesion may be a nonmalignant hypertrophy resulting from trauma.

226 In avian medicine, ultrasonography is primarily used for the diagnosis of abdominal disorders. Because the structure of the viscera can be clearly demonstrated, this is an excellent diagnostic tool in the search for abdominal tumors and other changes of the liver, kidneys, and reproductive tract. Even some cardiac changes can be identified. This method, for example, allows the imaging of eggs with no shell or soft-shelled eggs and the demonstration of pericardial effusion, ascites, and ovarian cysts, which is not possible using radiography. Moreover, it is possible to differentiate between hypertrophy of the heart and pericardial effusion; organ swellings caused by hyperplasia, hypertrophy, or abnormal contents; and tumors. Nevertheless, in most cases, as in mammals, the combination of radiographic and ultrasonographic examination is superior to the use of a single diagnostic method, because this enables the veterinarian to have a more precise picture of the disease process.

227 **(a)** In this illustration the subcutaneous ulnar vein is being punctured close to the elbow joint.

(b) This vein is often relatively small in diameter, thin walled, and very liable to hematoma formation. Bleeding can be controlled by a pressure swab, preferably soaked with ferric chloride.

(c) The central continuation of this ulnar vein, which becomes the basilic vein, can also be used near the axilla. Probably the best site for the collection of larger amounts of blood in most birds, although not in the ostrich (because of the danger of a fatal hematoma), is the right jugular vein. This vein is also not accessible in pigeons. The medial metatarsal vein situated on the medial aspect of the tarsometatarsus is easily accessible in many species, and, because of the more robust surrounding tissues, hematoma formation is less likely.

If very small quantities of blood (e.g., DNA sampling for sexing, diagnosis of disease, or establishing parentage) then a toenail (or claw) clip will suffice. However, strict cleanliness is essential because the sample may contain urates, feces, dirt, and desquamated cells and so invalidate the sample.

(d) When collecting blood a maximum of 1% (in healthy birds) of the body weight should only be withdrawn. When giving fluids intravenously a maximum of 20 ml/kg body weight can be given as a bolus injection over a period of 5 to 10 minutes.

228 **(a)** A distended abdomen in a bird of this age is usually caused by one or more of the following:
  • An enlarged liver or ascites
  • An enlarged intestinal tract
  • A retained yolk sac
(b) If the bird is presented with hepatomegaly and is a psittacine (or sometimes in the case

of some finch species), then papovavirus infection (budgerigar fledgling disease) is very likely. Enlargement of the intestinal tract resulting from ileus may be because of a noninfectious cause. This may be due to a variety of causes of mechanical obstruction (much more likely in older birds), a neurogenic etiology, or an infectious agent (bacterial or fungal, possibly *Candida*). Avian serositis, another cause of abdominal distension, is usually seen in older chicks and older birds.

Normally the (internal) yolk sac is absorbed within the first few days of life (in ostriches it lasts longer, approximately 8 days). Failure to absorb the yolk sac is usually caused by an infection via the umbilicus, which can be the result of a faulty incubation technique.

229 (a) The radiograph shows distinct signs of osteolysis of the proximal femoral diaphysis. Also, there is a suspicion of an increase in diameter of the femoral cortex surrounding this area compared with that of the opposite side. Furthermore, there is the impression that the head of the femur looks deformed. There is no sign of a "sunburst" effect or periostitis.
(b) This is possibly a benign bone tumor or tuberculosis. In line with the chronicity of this lesion the muscle masses surrounding both femur and tibiotarsus are noticeably reduced.

230 (a) This swelling is caused by an overinflated cervicoencephalic air sac, which may be bilateral or unilateral. This air sac is one of the many extensive sacculations of the infraorbital sinus. Overinflation of the cervicoencephalic air sac is possibly traumatic in origin, with the junction between this air sac and the suborbital chamber of the infraorbital sinus becoming stretched and overenlarged. The differential diagnosis is rupture of an air sac or skin emphysema.
(b) Besides careful palpation, diagnosis can be confirmed by radiography.
(c) A surgical procedure has been described for correction of this abnormality, but this method requires microsurgery involving up to ×25 magnification.
An alternative and much simpler method is to incise the skin/air sac, creating a fistula, and maintain this open for about 3 days. This reduces the air pressure within the ruptured and inflated part and allows the walls of the air sac to adhere together. The procedure does not require anesthesia and often produces good results.

Bibliography

Benyon PH, Forbes NA, Harcourt-Brown NH: *Manual of raptors, pigeons and water-fowl,* Ames, Iowa, 1996, Iowa State University Press.

Campbell TW: *Avian hematology and cytology,* Ames, Iowa 1988, Iowa State University Press.

Coles BH: *Avian medicine and surgery,* ed 2, Oxford, 1997, Blackwell Science.

Dorrestein GM: *Studies on pharmocokinetics of some antibacterial agents in homing pigeons (Columba livia),* Ph.D thesis, Utrecht, The Netherlands, 1986, University of Utrecht.

Forshaw JM, Cooper WT: *Parrots of the world,* Melbourne, Australia, 1989, Landsdowne Editions.

Fowler ME, ed: Special medicine: birds. In: *Zoo and wild animal medicine,* ed 3, London, WB Saunders.

Jordan FTW: *Poultry diseases,* London, 1990, Ballière Tindall.

King AS *Birds: their structure and function,* ed 2, London, 1984, Ballière Tindall.

King AS, McLelland J, eds: *Form and function in birds,* vols 1-4, London, 1979, Academic Press.

Krautwald ME et al: *Atlas of radiographic anatomy of birds,* Berlin, 1991, Verlag Paul Parey.

Lumeij JT: *A contribution to clinical investigative methods for birds, with special reference to the racing pigeon (Columba livia domestica),* PhD thesis, Utrecht, The Netherlands, 1987, University of Utrecht.

McLelland J: *A color atlas of avian anatomy,* Philadelphia, 1991, WB Saunders Philadelphia.

Orosz SE et al: *Avian surgical anatomy,* Philadelphia, 1992, WB Saunders.

Petrak ML: *Diseases of cage and aviary birds,* ed 2, Philadelphia, 1982, Lea & Febiger:

Redig PT et al, eds: *Raptor biomedicine,* Yorkshire, United Kingdom, 1993, Chiron.

Ritchie BW, Harrison GJ, Harrison LR: *Avian medicine: principles and application,* Lake Worth, Fla, 1994, Wingers Publishing.

Rosskopf JRWJ, Woerpel RW, eds: *Diseases of cage and aviary birds,* ed 3, Philadelphia, 1996, Lea & Febiger.

Rubel GA, Isenbugel E, Wolvekamp P: *Atlas of diagnostic radiology of exotic pets,* Philadelphia, WB Saunders.

Schubot R, Clubb S, Clubb K: *Psittacine aviculture,* Loxahatchee, Fla, 1992, Avicultural Breeding and Research Center.

Steiner CV, Davis RB: *Caged bird medicine: selected topics,* Ames, Iowa, 1981, Iowa State University Press.

Sturkie PD: *Avian physiology,* ed 4, New York, Springer Verlag.

Westerhof I: *Pituitary-adrenocortical function and glucocorticoid administration in pigeons (Columba livia domestica),* PhD thesis, Utrecht, The Netherlands, 1996, University of Utrecht.

Wobeser GA: *Diseases of wild waterfowl,* ed 2, New York, Plenum Press, 1997.

INDEX

200

Pantothenic acid deficiency
  hyperkeratosis caused by, 130
  malnutrition causing, 138
Papilloma-like growth involving
  rima glottis, 49, 152-153
Papillomas in canaries and finch-
  es, 144
Papillomaviruses, 30, 144
Papovavirus infection, 195
Parabuteo unicinctus, 74, 147
Parakeet, 17
Parakeratosis, dietary deficiency
  causing, 17, 138
Paralysis, 142
  flaccid, 188
Paramyxovirus infection
  group 3, 5, 131-132
  serotype group 1-pigeon, 145
Paramyxoviruses, 145
  group 3, vaccination for, in
    turkeys, 132
Parasites
  malarial, 56, 156
  in trachea, 154
Parasitic infections, 168
Parathyroid glands, enlargement
  of, 154
Paresis, 142
  of legs, 58, 157
Parrot(s), 20, 36, 52, 82
  Amazon; *see* Amazon parrot
  avulsion of beak in, 144
  cataracts in, 191
  diet for, 164
  grey, 26, 37, 76, 77, 109
    African, 10, 24, 28, 31, 44,
      48, 49, 51, 59, 64, 65, 71,
      73, 74, 89, 106, 112, 116,
      119, 134
    self-mutilation in, 37, 146
    Timneh, 32, 92, 144-145
  hanging, Philippine, 41
  metabolic bone disease in, 155
  mouth of, examination of, 188
  Neophema, group 3 paramyx-
    ovirus infection in, 5,
    131-132
  Pacheco's disease and, 131
  Pionus
    blue-headed, 38, 147
    feather cysts in, 150
  Platycercus, group 3 paramyx-
    ovirus infection in, 131
  red lored Amazon, 6

red shining, 10, 133
  restraint for, 188
  superb, 103
  tongues of, 143
  turquoise, 11, 35
  vasa, psittacine beak and
    feather disease in, 135
Passer domesticus, PMV 1-pigeon
  carried by, 145
Passeriformes
  "air sac mites" in, 154
  filariasis infection in, 174
  hatching in, 129
  hyperkeratosis in, 130
  trypanosomes in, 156
Pasteurellosis, 137
Patagonian conure, 97
Peach-faced lovebird, 41
Peafowl, PMV 1-pigeon in, 145
Pecten, 170
Pectoral muscles, atrophy of, 176
Pedicle, ligation of, 185
Peg, intramedullary, 183
Pendulous crop, treatment of,
  146
Penicillium spp., mycotic infec-
  tion caused by, 134
Perch, inability to, hyperkeratitis
  causing, 130
Perches, 159
  unhygienic or same size,
    pododermatitis caused
    by, 137
Peregrine falcon, 13
  blood uric acid levels in, 160
Periocular swelling, 60, 158
Peritonitis
  egg, 186
  egg yolk, 171
Pernis apivorus, 83, 169
Perosis, 155
Persistent feather sheaths, dietary
  deficiency causing, 17,
  138
Petroleum jelly for knemidocop-
  tic mange, 138
Phallus, pathologically extruded,
  30, 144
Pheasants, 63, 108
  PMV 1-pigeon in, 145
Philippine hanging parrot, 41
Phlebotomy for hemochromato-
  sis, 141
Phosphorus deficiency, 149

Phosphorus-calcium ratio, 164
  "angel wing" caused by, 135
Pigeon(s), 29, 34, 39, 40, 60, 61,
    80, 143
  Hippoboscids in, 132
  metabolic bone disease in, 155
  racing, 90
Pigeon pox virus, 140
Pigment colors of feathers, 129
Pigmentation, feather, *Aspergillus*
    infection causing, 134
Pins(pinning)
  during healing, 186
  intramedullary, 183
  removing, 189
Pionus menstruus, 38
Pionus parrot
  blue-headed, 38, 147
  feather cysts in, 150
Pipis, loss of foot in, 131
Plasma
  changes in, 171
  yellow, 171
Plasma protein values, total, 171
Plasmodium sp., 56, 156
  infection with, diagnosis of,
    157
Plaster casts, 156
Plates, bone, 183
Platycercus parrots, group 3
    paramyxovirus infec-
    tion in, 131
Plumage; *see also* Feathers(feath-
    ering)
  condition of, as indicator of
    health, 130
  disease and, 129
  factors responsible for, 129
  oil-soaked, cleaning of, 140
Pneumonia, 157
Podicipedidae, molting in, 129
Pododermatitis; *see*
    "Bumblefoot"
Poikilocytosis, 79, 168
Poisoning, 145; *see also*
    Intoxication
  algal, 137
  heavy metal, 150, 160-161
    hemoglobinemia and, 171
  lead, 136, 160-161
    diagnosis of, 168
    hematologic changes
      caused by, 79, 168
Polychromasia, 79, 168